MISSION
AFGHANISTAN

MISSION AFGHANISTAN

AN ARMY DOCTOR'S MEMOIR

BY ELIE PAUL COHEN

TRANSLATED BY JESSICA LEVINE

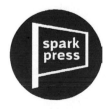

spark
press

Published by SparkPress, a BookSparks imprint,

A division of SparkPoint Studio, LLC

Tempe, Arizona, USA, 85281

www.gosparkpress.com

Published 2018

Printed in the United States of America

ISBN: 978-1-943006-65-6 (pbk)

ISBN: 978-1-943006-66-3 (e-bk)

Library of Congress Control Number: 2018940088

In memory of my father

CONTENTS

TRANSLATOR'S INTRODUCTION

Elie Paul Cohen was a civilian physician in his mid-fifties when the French Army asked him to become an emergency doctor liaison and travel to Afghanistan in order to report on medical techniques used there by British and American doctors.

Dr. Cohen was the man for the job for several reasons. Born and educated in France, he had obtained British citizenship after working in Britain for the National Health Service for ten years, while commuting back to Paris to maintain a part-time medical practice there. He also was an experienced emergency doctor, or *urgentiste*, which made him perfectly qualified. Here an explanation is in order. In the United States and the UK, the men and women working in ambulances are usually paramedics who are trained to implement diagnostic and lifesaving techniques that will extend a patient's life until transferred to the hospital. But they have far less medical training than physicians. In France, however, ambulances are staffed by doctors with special training in emergency medicine. With his knowledge of the health care systems of both France and the UK, his ability to speak both languages, and his training in emergency medicine, Dr. Cohen was particularly suited to work alongside British and American colleagues in military medicine.

Once in Afghanistan, Dr. Cohen quickly integrated himself into the routines of Role 3 Hospital at Camp Bastion. However, his position and point of view remained unique. Being a soldier is necessarily a defining experience; becoming a soldier in middle age, when you were anti-militarist in your youth, is an extraordinary, even surreal one. Undertaking a solo mission under those circumstances, Dr. Cohen became the quintessential outsider, an emissary into a very strange and unusual world. That status was reinforced by other factors. First, he was the only Frenchman at Camp Bastion. Also, while going through his training, Dr. Cohen was not attached to any specific unit. Finally, unlike his colleagues, he had worked as a civilian doctor for thirty years and was not a career military man. Thus he brought to the job the perspective of someone who questioned war, and this war in particular, recognizing both its necessity and its heartbreaking futility. It is this outsider point of view that gives Dr. Cohen's narrative its poignancy and power.

—*Jessica Levine*

1.
LEAVING FOR AFGHANISTAN

Summer of 2011. Roissy Charles de Gaulle Airport. It's late afternoon. The airport seems abnormally empty for this time of the year. It's hot and humid outside. The atmosphere is charged with electricity, like a sky threatening a storm.

I'm standing in front of one of the boarding counters in the group of soldiers I'm traveling with. Like them, I'm wearing a uniform in the colors of the French Army. A cotton T-shirt, a jacket and pants too heavy for the season, printed with multicolored motifs, shades of khaki green and brown evoking foliage that are supposed to help camouflage us. It looks more suitable for wooded or mountainous zones than for the beige of the desert where I'll be stationed. My green wool socks look like the ones I use when I go climbing high in the mountains. As for shoes, when I found that the ones the army had provided were too stiff, I bought some myself on the advice of a pal in the Special Forces. A soldier walks a lot and has to take care of his feet, so I invested in a pair of Blackwalk shoes that are supple, ventilated, and suitable for mountainous and desert terrain.

1

My kit is reduced to a strict minimum. A backpack, another bag over my shoulder, packed as lightly as possible because on the ground where I'm going, I'll have to be mobile. I'm taking extras of everything: two spare T-shirts and three extra pairs of socks, two bath towels, my toiletry bag, my laptop computer and USB sticks loaded with books, music, and movies. I have also packed fingerless shooting gloves, sunglasses, a switchblade knife, and earplugs for when I'll be in a helicopter. They gave me a gas mask in case of a chemical attack—an unlikely eventuality. As it's rather bulky, I've attached it to the outside of my backpack. I had to cut my hair very short. It's usually on the long side, so that's a change for me. For a guy who was an anti-militarist rebel in his youth and has always kept himself apart from groups, I've gotten myself into a surreal situation. . . .

It is 7:30 p.m. as I stand on line for registration. Destination Dushanbe in Tajikistan, a French base in Central Asia and the entryway to Afghanistan. We're scheduled to make a brief stop in Cyprus beforehand. For some reason that escapes me, we're leaving from a civilian airport although the plane belongs to the Air Force.

Delayed by traffic, I've barely had time to kiss Clara, my partner, who insisted on accompanying me to the airport. A complicated goodbye because, once there, anything can happen. We are both aware of this without spelling it out.

I'm leaving for what the military calls a "theater of operations." War is like a drama played live on a stage.

"I have to admit, you look good in a soldier's uniform, Doctor Elie," she says with her typical tenderness and kind humor. "In fact, you look good in everything. You could wear a dinner jacket and football shorts and you'd still be chic. A real Don Juan!"

"Now you're pulling my leg!"

Clara is a beautiful brunette with blue eyes unchanged by the passing of years. After having gone to the Beaux-Arts to study painting and decorative arts for interior design, she worked first as a journalist then as a talented artistic director in the luxury industry. Many of my friends envy me for having a partner who's both smart and sexy. I was finishing my medical studies when we first crossed paths in the cafeteria of the hospital where I worked at the time. She was visiting a family member who was hospitalized in the pulmonology department. I became attached to this young widow and her baby, Paul, whom I would raise as my son.

As often happens, time and life events have made our love more fragile. And then the temptation of a young British woman, Laura, complicated the picture. I'd met her three years earlier, in London, where she was taking a class on pain management that I was teaching at the university. She asked me to be her thesis director. Feeling a mutual attraction, and not wanting to mix my professional and personal lives, I'd refused.

But a couple of years later, Laura passed through Paris and contacted me. Young and pretty, pretending to be sweet and innocent, she did everything to tempt me into an affair. In the tense context of my leaving for Afghanistan and my home situation, I almost crossed the threshold. An ambiguous relationship began between us.

Clara learned about it, of course, when her feminine intuition was confirmed by a text message she happened to discover on my cell phone. After passing through anger and feelings of betrayal, she was led by her natural compassion to forgive me on the condition I broke with Laura. Which I did. My military mission came at a key moment in my story with Clara. This forced parenthesis was a kind of test, at the crossroads of her path and mine.

And here we are, standing in the concourse at Charles de Gaulle airport like a couple of teenagers who can't bear to part.

"You could have done something else for your vacation besides leaving for war," she says. "What a weird idea, really, and just like you! Above all, be careful. Paul and I want to see you again."

"Don't worry, Clara. You know this whole business is just a product of circumstance."

"Circumstance that could turn into a cruel destiny, if you die over there. What a crazy story you invented for your parents and your sister to justify your long absence. I wonder if they believed it!"

"It's to protect them, you know that!" I say. My elderly parents might not be able to handle my going to a war zone.

"In the meantime, I'll be the one to give them the bad news, if there is any."

"I'll come back!"

Watching her leave and disappear at the end of the boarding area, I tell myself that we're acting out a bad script I can only hope to survive.

∼

Night begins to fall. After registration, we pass through customs and airport security with civilians bound for other flights. In line, a noncom in his mid-thirties turns to me, smiling. Stocky, with a moustache and a face lined by experience, he belongs to that class of professional military men who have known every kind of country. "Captain," he says, "you should remove your belt. You don't need to wear it around your waist with the summer uniform."

In the army, function and experience prevail over rank. I do as he advises.

"You're going where in Afghanistan?" he asks me.

"To Camp Bastion, in Helmand Province," I answer. Helmand is in the south of the country, toward Pakistan and Iran.

"But isn't that a British zone?"

"That's right. I'm an emergency doctor. They're sending me on a liaison mission."

"I see. Unusual for a doctor in the French Army! That's a region where the fighting is hard and intense. Have you already been in a war zone, doc?"

"No! You know, I'm not a career military doctor. It's by coincidence that I've ended up in the army."

"By coincidence!" he answers, smiling. "How can anyone go to war by coincidence? You surely have reasons you can't share. I hope you at least went through some training?"

"Yes, but relatively brief, an 'acculturation,' as they call it in the army. I spent time in Lorient, with the Marine Commandos, and six weeks in Djibouti. I topped it off with a physical training program with a coach to get back in shape, then I spent time at a shooting club in the Paris area practicing with handguns and assault weapons with help from people in the Special Forces."

Our conversation continues. I learn that he is, as I suspected, a career military man in the marine infantry, and that in fifteen years he has gone everywhere the French Army is present. Africa, in particular. This is the first time he is leaving for Afghanistan with his fellow soldiers; he's going to the Bagram area. Our destinies have crossed in this airport and this plane, and they will separate once we arrive in Tajikistan.

∼

You can feel the tension growing in this group of soldiers leaving for war. Consciously or unconsciously, and depending on their level of experience, they know they are going to live through a dangerous and unusual adventure, one they might not return from. Whether wounded or safe and sound, they will come out having undergone a deep metamorphosis.

While waiting to board, I drink an orange juice in the cafeteria.

It gives me the chance to get into a conversation with three technicians in the maintenance crew for the air force. It's the second time they'll be serving in Afghanistan. They're traveling to Kandahar where part of the French Air Force is based. Unlike the noncom of the navy troops, they have never been directly involved in combat.

Once there, I'll realize that not all soldiers are equally in danger in a war, for their level of exposure depends on their function. A maintenance technician risks his life less than a fighter in the Special Forces. Yet this secondary kind of service is useful and complementary, because an army cannot run without strong logistics. I'll soon understand the specificity and complexity of deploying troops for the Afghan conflict, a counter-insurgency war without a true front line, where an attack can spring out of anywhere.

After boarding, I find myself in the section of the airplane reserved for officers. The flight crew belongs to the air force. The hostesses are pretty and friendly. In spite of their kind smiles, I read in their eyes, so full of compassion, that our arrival will be a descent into hell. I'm sitting next to three lieutenant colonels. There's no space to stretch out my legs. And I'm going to have to travel ten to twelve hours in this position. After having greeted my travel companions cordially, I withdraw back into my bubble, concentrating on the objectives of my mission. The atmosphere in the plane is meditative. Before turning off my cell, I send a couple of loving text messages to Clara and Paul.

Suddenly I'm thinking again about Laura. Before authorizing my deployment to Afghanistan, the military intelligence service, called DPSD for Direction de la Protection et de la Sécurité de la Défense,[1] inquired into almost all of my contacts going back several years, my own family included, and warned me to be prudent

---

1 The name of this organization was changed to DRSD for Direction du Renseignement et de la Sécurité de la Défense in October 2016. (Trans. note)

with that woman. Why did they share their doubts about her? I don't know if they were motivated by some spy-type paranoia or factual evidence, but it's true that as soon as you start working with the army, the most improbable scenarios can take on meaning. But maybe the DPSD is wrong and the case is simply that she's not the first student to want to sleep with her professor—a story with no resolution.

It's past midnight. The plane will soon take off. Wanting to understand the nature of my mission better, I skim a book about the geopolitics of the Afghan conflict, while listening through headphones to "Over the Rainbow" on my cell, superbly sung by Eva Cassidy. Maybe it's the song affecting me, but suddenly I have a bizarre feeling, as though I were floating between dream and reality. Little by little, my thoughts drift away from my book and I begin to travel into my past. Memories parade by in my head. . . .

2.
THE TWO ELIES

How did I end up in Central Asia, six thousand kilometers away from home, in the hell of war, in this land of Afghanistan, so harsh and mysterious, almost enchanting? Adding to the strangeness of my situation, I have the impression, perhaps not justifiable, that I am only one of a few Jews serving in the NATO troops, an undesirable, unbelieving infidel in this Islamic so-called *res publica*, a republic that exists in name only and in its flag.

Here, contrast rules. Cell phones coexist with customs from the Middle Ages. Violence and spirituality commune, as though God and the Devil had met here to come to terms with each other in one of the most seismically active zones of our beautiful planet. From the eternal snows of the Hindu Kush in the north to the infernal desert of the Helmand in the south, nature often proves to be hostile.

Reflecting this region, the many ethnicities that populate it are tough and inured to hardship, for they have survived poverty, a lack of hygiene, illiteracy, drugs, and a war that has raged for over thirty years. The fighters are resilient, accustomed to precarious living conditions, and familiar with every corner of their mountains and deserts. Modest peasants by day, some of them will turn into formidable warriors at night.

All of this seems so far from what we French call *la douce France*—sweet France—which is never satisfied with its lot, or the United Kingdom, my second homeland. Yet, in the last century, these two nations also suffered through two world wars. I myself was born in Algeria toward the end of the 1950s, during this former colony's war for independence. The region had been an Ottoman province for three centuries before becoming a French colony in 1830, then a French *département* or province in 1848. The French Army, composed mostly of conscripts mobilized to maintain order, became bogged down in a conflict pervaded by a tribal element that is now often forgotten. In certain ways, the Afghan guerillas of today can be compared to those of the FLN, the Algerian National Liberation Front, except that religion wasn't a factor in the Algerian war for independence as it has been in Afghanistan, where religion is used as an ideological pretext. The Afghan *mujahideen*, who fought the Soviet forces from 1979 to 1989, were using a name already used by the Algerian *fellagha*. In Arab, the word *mujahideen* means resistant or militant.

~

I have no memory of Algeria because my family left shortly after my birth. But, in thinking about it again, I realize clearly that war has always, in some subliminal manner, been part of my life. Like many people of my generation, I was raised amid memories of 1914-18 and 1939-45. As a child, I rarely visited a home where a grandfather, father, or uncle hadn't been mobilized in one of those terribly bloody conflicts. I was viscerally affected by Nazism and the history of the Holocaust. Additionally, there was the creation of the State of Israel and its conflicts with the Arab world.

I don't have much information about the origins of either my paternal or maternal families. It's true that over the course of centuries, the Jewish people have often undergone forced migrations, and it's not easy to retrace the path of each one of them. Ever since the destruction of its kingdom by the Romans two thousand years ago, the Diaspora spread into different areas of the world and has never stopped expanding, from the Middle East to Europe, from Asia to North Africa. Expelled from France, England, and Spain in the Middle Ages, then subjected to pogroms in Russia and to Nazi extermination, the Jews have finally regrouped in the United States and Israel.

A genealogist friend of mind told me that my paternal grandfather, Elie, had ancestors from Palestine who settled in the Maghreb in northwest Africa. The reasons for this move, if it did take place, remain mysterious. The ancestors of my paternal grandmother, Esther, would have arrived in Algeria after having been chased out of Spain at the moment of the Inquisition established by the Catholic Queen Isabella in 1492. On my mother's side, the family origins of my grandmother, Marie, and my grandfather, Abraham, supposedly go back to Central Europe. Maybe they belonged to those Jews of the Rhine valley who traded with North Africa. The trade routes would then have led them to settle there, but I can't know for sure. In short, all of this is conjecture. A wandering Jew with universal views, I'm of mixed Oriental Sephardic and Occidental Ashkenazi heritage. As I've always preferred being open to the world over staying in the ghetto, this combination suits me.

～

In Algeria, we lived facing the Mediterranean, in a little fishing village, at that time called Nemours, located near the Moroccan border. It apparently had this odd name in homage to the French aristocrat, Louis d'Orléans, duc de Nemours. Before the Arabs and the Ottomans, the Romans had called it Ad Fratres. Today it has been rebaptized Ghazaouet. According to the ancients, the countryside was magnificent then, and, as far back as can be remembered, people fished there for sardines and anchovies.

My paternal family formed a clan. Elie, my grandfather, was the patriarch. I bear his name. I've always heard that he had a special affection for me. In 1916, he was twenty years old. Recruited into the *Deuxième Zouaves*—the regiment from the French African colonies—he struggled by the side of his brothers-in-arms in the cold, the mud, the violence, and anguish of the trenches at Verdun and in the north of France. The Great War affected his health. He was lucky enough to return wounded only in the Achilles' tendon by a shell fragment. He was hit there on November 11, 1918, the last day of the war, at eleven o'clock in the morning, just one hour before the official end of the war.

Like him, many men from the colonies, coming from different cultures and faiths, bravely fought for France, the mother country that often betrayed them. What remains of all of it?

In my grandfather's case, fragile health, a military cross, and memories that marked him deeply. When he returned, he married Esther before leaving for yet another war, this time in Rif, Morocco. They would have nine children, three of whom would die young, probably from infectious diseases. Six others would remain, two girls and four boys, including my father, Lucien. In order to feed his family, my grandfather learned the tailor's trade and opened a shop. My father, as an adolescent, followed in his footsteps.

Two of my grandfather's sons would be mobilized during the

Algerian war. Sensing that the winds were changing and that the situation of the French in Algeria had become difficult, the entire clan left and settled in Paris shortly after my birth. My grandfather Elie must have been deeply marked by these events, for he died shortly afterwards, and the family he had cemented together soon burst apart. I'd just reached my first birthday. I never really knew him. As for pictures of him, I've only seen two. In one of them, on his veteran's card, he must be thirty years old. The other was taken shortly before his death. Both young and old, he has the same gaze, reflecting the depth of his soul which, in spite of life's wounding, was able to remain intact until the end.

I've often thought about him these past years and felt his benevolent presence. At first, I didn't know why. At present, I understand a little better. What a strange similarity exists between us, the two Elies. He who had already associated with the British during World War I, and I, deployed today by their side, in a world war of a third kind. History works in cycles of eternal return.

Visibly impressed by the British, he often spoke to my father of their legendary composure, of how they continued to shave in the trenches while the bombs fell around them, as if nothing special were happening. He had a deep respect for them that he surely transmitted to me, because when I became an adult, I went so far as to settle in the United Kingdom and obtain British citizenship.

The extreme situation I've landed in at present has clearly brought us closer together. This transgenerational thread plays a key role in the unexpected trial I'm going through. Bit by bit, an interior dialogue has taken hold inside me, almost as though I were a medium and my grandfather were guiding me. I have the bizarre impression that his invisible, almost paranormal presence is protecting me. It helps me avoid traps and make good choices. Maybe this sensation is only imaginary, but its effect on me is positive. When I find myself deployed with the French and British forces in another war, it helps me backtrack along Ariadne's thread, in order to understand how I've reached this point.

If I'm here today, it's because I have a double debt to pay to both my grandfather and the army. When I was twenty, I was anti-militarist and avoided military service. If my grandfather Elie, whose loyalty to France was absolute, had been alive at the time, he would have been furious and disappointed with me. Would I have acted as I did if he'd been there to witness my rebellion? Perhaps I would have all the same. My very nature and my education probably also have something to do with it. Ironically, I'm in the army now.

Insecurity, ambivalence, and adaptability have marked my life from the beginning. As soon as I was born, I was uprooted by war and forced to leave my place of birth, Algeria, in order to head for my country, France. There my family had to start over from scratch. This exodus and our arrival in Paris was a kind of immigration, because at the beginning, the way others looked at us made us doubt that we belonged to the national community. We were French, but we had arrived from North Africa. Then finally life resumed its course, and we progressively interiorized the social codes and culture of our new milieu.

Transplanted to the streets of Paris, far from the blue of the Mediterranean and the perfumes of North Africa, I always felt close to the weak and the foreign, like those populations that are today displaced by war and poverty. Their no man's land has always been mine, too.

My sister and I grew up in the working-class areas of Paris, where we went to school and learned the values of the French Republic—liberty, equality, brotherhood—alongside the immigrant children of the time. The kids came from Spanish, Italian, and Portuguese families or they had parents from Maghreb, called *pieds-noirs* (black feet) for those French born in Algeria before its independence. In spite of the tensions and the occasional fights, all of us boys and girls mostly adapted to the system. I should add, however, that in Europe in the Sixties, extremism, fundamentalism, racism, and anti-Semitism, although they existed, did not govern thinking the way they do today, when immigration and terrorism have increased the scope and intensity of these problems. As the end of World War II and its atrocities still felt close, few people in Western societies dared to call into question the right to difference that everyone speaks about at present.

Mixed in with the insecurity caused by our uprooting and the adaptability needed for successful integration, there was ambivalence about which group I belonged to. Here my Jewish roots complicated the picture. As a child, I felt I was from neither Algeria nor France. Matters weren't helped by the conversations among the adults in my family around me, my father, mother, uncles and aunts, still traumatized by World War II, the Holocaust, and the recent events in Algeria that had just taken their lives apart in a deep way. Doubt about everything took root in me when I was little, and I initially took refuge in what my immediate environment offered me—Judaism and Israel. Later, as an adolescent, I gradually detached myself from these havens, in order to replace them with other interests, such as sports, music, poetry, and girls, of course.

At home, we remained united when confronted with difficulties. My father was employed by the RATP, the Paris Métro system. In Algeria, he had served in the French Navy before starting to fish for anchovies and sardines on trawlers, at night, by lamplight. From being a sailor on the Mediterranean to a ticket puncher under the streets of Paris—what a nosedive!

His modest pay was enough to put dinner on the table. It should be added that my mother, Raymonde, could make a feast out of not much. Intellectual by nature and a hairdresser by economic necessity, she hardly practiced this trade that she was forced to learn, and she dedicated herself almost completely to our education. Take a father, a mother, and their two children, put them in a tiny apartment, add a lot of love and sacrifice, stir gently over a low fire for several years, and with a little luck you'll get a family that more or less stays the course.

When it came to doing stupid things, however, I did my share. I was a difficult adolescent, a rebel who hung out in the streets with my buddies or, later on, in the cafés near my high school. My mother would come to get me and drag me back home in the days I was still young enough for her to do so. I realize now that she was in the right because some of my pals from the period spent years of their lives in prison or have already died as a result of addiction to hard drugs.

Fortunately, I was lucky enough to meet extraordinary educators. Intuitively, I knew not to cross the fateful red line on the other side of which lay the land of no return. A very strong survival instinct guided me and guides me still along the front zones of Afghanistan, where I've been deployed. The army must know this, since it was the one to sentence me to the galleys. People have often told me I was playing Russian roulette. Personally, I don't think so, or if so, only because I had to. Necessity creating its own reality.

If I'm a survivor, I also owe it to sports and music. These two provided axes that have marked out my life's path and have enabled me to meet remarkable beings. In spite of their meager means, my parents always saw to developing our talents. As soon as I learned to walk, whenever I saw a piano, I'd make sure to go tap on it. My father noticed my attraction to this instrument. He himself was crazy about Louis Armstrong.

At home, we listened to records in mono on an old, light gray Teppaz. All kinds got played: jazz, classical, and pop. I can still see myself at four years old, sitting on the ground, leaning over the turntable, playing Edith Piaf singing *"L'Homme à la moto"* over and over again, or the introduction of Tchaikovsky's *Concerto n°1*, interpreted by Giörgy Cziffra on piano. I was literally fascinated, as though hypnotized by the voice of this tremendous singer and the famous melody in the first measures of Tchaikovsky's magnificent piece of music.

When I was almost seven, my parents enrolled me in a *conservatoire municipal*, a music school for kids and teenagers, to study music theory and then piano. I knocked around as a dilettante for a few years. For one thing, we didn't have a piano at home for lack of space. I'd practice on paper keyboards or occasionally on a neighbor's instrument. When I began grammar school, my father finally bought us a study piano with a tilting keyboard, perfect for our tiny lodgings. Everything changed at that point. A new dynamic started, I could finally give music form on my own instrument. The pieces of the puzzle began to fall into place. And I would soon make an acquaintance that would be decisive for my life.

I was thirteen years old when Simone, a pianist with the Paris opera, came into my life. She arrived as a new piano teacher at the music school where I hung out. She was a great musician. First prize in piano at the Conservatoire National Supérieur de Musique in Paris, she had worked with the best choreographers and dancers of the time: Serge Lifar, Roland Petit, Michel Renault, Mikhaïl Baryshnikov, and Rudolf Nureyev. The electroshock worked. Step by step, over several years, with an artist's rigor and a mother's patience, she disciplined me, taught me how to work, and transformed this adolescent rebel into a professional musician. She marked my destiny in a positive fashion by preventing me from going up in smoke before I'd even started my life. We remained close until her death. Without her presence, I never would have become a musician or even a doctor. Thanks to her, these two professions, which a priori had nothing to do with each other, became linked in an unexpected way.

Once I had my high school diploma in my pocket, I was attracted to medicine, but my father wasn't Rockefeller. Here my mentor Simone intervened a second time. "You're a musician, Elie, I'll help you pass the exam to become a music teacher for the city of Paris. You'll need a year to prepare. It's within your reach. In the meantime, complete your education by enrolling in the musicology department and find odd jobs to get by."

"And medicine, Simone?"

"You'll come back to it later. You're gifted for showbiz, and you have the looks for it, too. Earn some money composing songs for others, since you enjoy that. You'll see, one day it will help you finance your medical studies."

That's pretty much how things went. Simone was certainly very lucid, even clairvoyant. A year later, I was a music teacher by day and a nightclub pianist at night, while pursuing studies in musicology. After I established a working base, my next task was to penetrate the recording industry. Life's chance encounters helped me. Very soon I met the right people, including a music publisher who would be important for me. Two years later, I was composing for advertising that was being broadcast. Then I landed a job as an artistic director in the French branch of CBS Records. Everything was going my way, money was coming in, girls liked me, but something was missing.

That "something" was medicine, which in my eyes symbolized a humanitarian and spiritual quest. That ideal certainly helped me survive the shark-infested world that I moved in during that period. I loved music, but I didn't like the entertainment world; all of its tinsel and marketing struck me as phony. Too many drugs there, too. As an adolescent, I'd seen so many of my friends destroyed by substance abuse that I wasn't about to let myself fall into that trap. In reaction, I did a lot of sports, while figuring out how to extricate myself. When someone suggested I should be a singer, a new career path was open to me, but I held back to avoid the limelight, as my only objective was to stay in the shadows and accumulate enough money to pay for my studies. Of course I didn't share my plans with anyone. In this manner, I stayed afloat in this environment for a few years.

I was twenty-six when the conditions were right for me to make a change. I'd earned enough money from my music royalties to stop for a while and try to realize my dream, until then inaccessible, of becoming a doctor. I had to get out of the entertainment world very fast, because it's not easy to leave this milieu where business is based on exchanged favors and debts. In the space of two months, I literally disappeared without leaving an address, in the style of "take the money and run." A little holdup, fair enough, because I had a right to the money I'd earned honestly with the sweat of my compositions. But folks in show business don't like to lose one of their own without getting a return on their investment. It therefore wasn't in my interest to step back into the system. The door was now closed for me—and no regrets! I've never gone back, or rather, when I did, it was much later and in experimental music, which was less commercial.

And then, I entered a long tunnel. It was to be expected; my medical studies were difficult. I had to leave my comfortable apartment for a student's room where I lived meagerly, like a Spartan, financing my studies with my music royalties and shifts as a hospital nurse.

Sports helped me through this, too. I discovered boxing through Charley, another remarkable connection, and took to it. Although kind by nature, I had, stemming from anxiety, a violent streak that I learned to channel thanks to this noble art. Toward the end of the 1950s, Charley had been a professional middleweight champion in

France. As he was well-known in Europe during his career, the movies came after him. Luchino Visconti, having noticed his blue eyes and his Brando boxer physique, had invited him to appear in *Rocco and His Brothers.*

Having later become a trainer, Charley taught this discipline at university. With him I practiced this sport as a university boxer for eight years. I'd go to the boxing club several times a week, in rain, snow, or wind, even after a night shift at the hospital. It boosted my energy; I no longer suffered from lack of sleep and could swing into my day as usual. He turned me into a French university middleweight runner-up. He was a profoundly human being, a teacher and a friend whom the Grim Reaper would cut down too early.

~

When I look back at the road traveled, I see a true obstacle course, similar, in certain regards, to the one that has led me to Afghanistan. Life is also a war without a front that one wages above all for oneself. Zero risk does not exist, although we may have been led to believe otherwise. In my case, I didn't have a choice; when I chose medicine, there would be no going back. In the same way, I am now meant to complete my mission as an army doctor and to return safe and sound.

Strangely, I've always lived according to a rhythm out of sync with others. In medical school, I was eight years older than the other students who had just graduated. I'm now almost twenty-five years older, on average, than the soldiers I'm deployed with. This gap finally became second nature to me. I became used to it to the point that I learned how to turn it into an asset, for it forced me to question and surpass myself. It hardened me.

I don't know whether the army chose well when it cast me as a soldier bound for Afghanistan, but it certainly evaluated my endurance for long journeys and my taste for extreme situations. In the meantime, I'm in this Afghan quagmire, and I have to make good. I remember what my friend Octave, one of those shadow heroes who fought in World War II, said: "You see, Elie, in the Middle East as in Patton's army, I took on war like a sport. Thinking like that helped me get through it." It's my turn now to try to do that, but it's a funny sport all the same. Death or disability may be waiting at the end of the path. If given a choice, I'd prefer to die. In any case, when I think about it again, this story started in a rather burlesque fashion. . . .

3.
REBEL

Three years earlier. September 2008. I'm still living in the United Kingdom where I work as a physician, but I'm thinking of making a change. I could return to France but I'm seriously considering Australia, which has been interested in recruiting me into their health system. On this particular day, I'm in Paris where I have an appointment at the Ordre des Médecins, or General Medical Council, in order to bring my professional dossier up to date after having spent ten years in Her Majesty the Queen's country.

Times have changed, but as I step into the Haussmannian building where I'm expected, I can't help reflecting that this institution took shape during the Second World War, under the Vichy government. I therefore remain rather reserved when I have to deal, either directly or from a distance, with this regulatory organization representing the professional interests of physicians.

A staff member receives me. He must be in his fifties. Skinny, with gray hair that's been cut very short, he wears big eyeglasses behind which radiates a clear and empathetic glance contrasting with the apparent dryness of his character. Sitting behind his desk, he seems ready and willing to listen.

"Your dossier is in order. I see you're an emergency physician. With a complete profile and international experience. Dual French and British nationality. In fact, why do you have dual nationality—you were born in France, right?"

"Yes, that's correct, but I finished my internship in London, where I subsequently practiced medicine for many years. For practical and administrative reasons, my British colleagues and friends advised me to adopt British nationality. They helped me with the procedure, and I took the plunge."

"From what I can see, it was also the English who financed some of your studies in emergency medicine in France. That's unusual!"

"Yes, it happened in the context of continuing education. They were interested in how the SAMU runs," I said, referring to the French pre-hospital emergency service, "and they financed my study leave so I could get my diploma in emergency medicine in France."

"They've lagged behind us for years," he said, referring to the fact that at the time the UK health system was in need of improvement. "But I can see from what you're telling me that they're updating their program."

"Yes, unlike what you may have heard about the National Health Service on this side of the Channel, the evaluation and training of their physicians is beginning to work."

"The tabloids were unjustly hard on our emergency services after the death of Lady Di. I see that our favorite rivals are making progress and catching up in this domain. We should wake up, if we don't want to move backwards." He pauses, then adds, "At present, I have to leave you. My next appointment has arrived, and I don't have the time to take your professional dossier down to the diploma office. Could you do it for me? Goodbye, and good luck!"

The guy doesn't know just how on target he is with that last wish, because when it comes to luck, I'm really going to need it!

〜

Relaxed and satisfied with the meeting, I calmly head down the staircase leading to the diploma office while I glance through my dossier, which I've never had access to before. The future seems luminous, without any apparent clouds. But it's too good to be true! Suddenly, I land on a key document I wasn't expecting to find there. The original of my military medical record. I'm reading this document for the first time in my life when I freeze on the staircase. *Damn!* I think. *The defiant psychopath described in here isn't anything like me. Even if I was coming out of a wild, Rimbaud-like adolescence, even if I did a bunch of stupid things to avoid the army, this still isn't me. Now I'm in a real stew as a doctor! If the Australian recruiters see this, my possibilities for going there could be compromised. Come to think of it, what is my military past doing in my civilian professional dossier anyway?*

I consider removing it, then hesitate when an internal voice, which I associate for some reason with my paternal grandfather, calls to me, "Be careful, Elie, don't do it! There are surely copies of it elsewhere."

I feel destabilized, suddenly projected many years back in time. Coincidence or fate? The events of an earlier era parade before my eyes . . .

〜

I'm twenty years old, rebelling against everything and especially against myself. Medicine is still far in the future. My Eldorado is songwriting. I'm trying to penetrate the music and recording world. In the meantime, I get by doing odd jobs. In France, at the end of the seventies, although military service is obligatory and lasts a year, the atmosphere isn't militaristic. The wars in Algeria and Vietnam, the Beat generation, hippies, Bob Dylan, The Beatles, and finally May '68 in France have left their mark on the younger generation. A perfume of Peace and Love still floats in the air.

Darkening the picture is the fact that, during the Second World War, my parents and their family lived under the discriminatory laws passed by the Vichy government and applied to the *Israélites*, as Jews were called at the time. Luckily, while my parents were living in North Africa, the American landing of 1942 helped them avoid deportation. Then there was the exodus of the *pieds-noirs*, the Israeli-Arab conflict, and the openly pro-Arab politics of France that began with the Six Day War. During my entire childhood, I thus harbored feelings of defiance toward my own country, France. With a young person's simplistic view of things, I was still far from understanding the complexity and subtleties of geopolitics.

At twenty, the age of conscription, I knew that the army's pre-enlistment selection process involved three days during which the intellectual and physical capacities of conscripts were tested. Next would come an assignment to a military corps that wasn't always best suited to one's abilities. When I was called up, I didn't have to be convinced to do anything and everything possible to get out of serving in the army. And that's what happened.

∼

It's morning, and I arrive ready to put on a show in order to get thrown out. I don't want to blow it. I've been preparing for several weeks. A student friend of mine from medical school gave me some speed that I took last night. I've never taken amphetamines before and was hoping I wouldn't sleep and would be overexcited. They've made me wired. What a stupid thing to do, now that I think about it!

From the beginning, I do the opposite of what they ask me to.

I answer the questions on the tests any which way. During the projection of a film of military propaganda, I start shouting, "This is bullshit, it's all lies," which provokes the beginning of an uprising in my group. Suddenly, in spite of myself, I'm an undesirable leader. A furious officer threatens to incorporate me immediately into a disciplinary battalion. I tell him to fuck off! I'm acting like an antisocial borderline personality, and I'm doing it with the energy of total despair. At the end of the three days, having stumbled into the trap I've set for myself, I inevitably end up at the military psychiatrist's.

Coincidence or destiny, one or the other will come into play.

I'm sitting in the waiting room. There are three of us future conscripts. In order of arrival, I should be the second one called. The guy sitting to my left feels like talking. He addresses me.

"I've been observing you for the past three days. You want to be declared unfit?"

"Yeah, I'd like that. In any case, that's what I'm trying for!"

"Listen! I'll go first. There are two doors with a psychiatrist behind each one. I'll take the one on the right. When it's your turn, you do the same thing. That doctor is willing to declare guys unfit. He already knows my case because he knows my family. Good luck!"

~

When it's my turn, the other door opens. At that moment I have a survival reflex. I turn to my neighbor on the right. "Go ahead! I'll wait," I said. He accepts with a nod, and a few minutes later I enter through the lucky door.

The psychiatrist has a cold expression behind his round eyeglasses. But as I'm thinking he might be won over to my cause, I give it my all. My conviction makes me more persuasive and he's understanding.

"You don't want to serve and you're playacting, right? I assure you, you're not the only one in that situation nowadays. What kind of work do you do?"

"Musician. I just got offered a job as music teacher for the City of Paris. If I don't take it immediately, I run the risk of losing it. I have to earn a living, I come from a working class family. I don't have a choice!"

"I understand. You don't look like an idiot. You're lucky, I'm in a good mood today. I'll find the right way to formulate your case."

∼

Like many young people of my generation, I wouldn't join the army. Happy that I'd reached my objective, a load off my shoulder, I was far from imagining that, one day many years later, this file once forgotten by the French Republic would float back up out of nowhere. Here I am now with this baby in my arms, standing alone on the big staircase at the General Medical Council, trying to decide what would be the best thing to do. Am I looking at the result of a normal procedure or a bomb they've intentionally left in my professional record? Or is it the consequence of simple negligence on the part of some busy bee who, after verifying it, should normally have sent it back to the army?

The woman in the diploma office receives me with a smile.

"Hello, Doctor, you're bringing in your professional dossier yourself, that's unusual!"

"I know, it was your colleague's idea. But there's a problem."

"Which is?"

"I found here something that looks like the original of my military record. Shouldn't it be in the army's archives?"

"Maybe. I myself am a veteran, and I find that peculiar. But after all, what's the problem? It was years ago, and military service is no longer obligatory."

A veteran, what a strange coincidence, I think.

"Take a look at it and you'll see that it would bother you, too, if you were in my shoes!"

She glances at it.

"Indeed, the psychiatrist of the time gave you quite a diagnosis! You were a student in medicine at the time of the pre-enlistment assessment?"

"No, I was starting a career in music, and I didn't yet know that I would go to medical school a few years later, even though that was my dream."

"It's rather embarrassing to have a stain like this on your civilian record. Given what I know about the military world, the only way to resolve this problem is to approach the army's health service."

"You think so?"

"Yes, Doctor, only the army can ask the General Medical Council to return your record to them."

"Why shouldn't I just destroy it now?"

"Not in front of me! It's too late, you should have done it in the staircase."

"I thought of doing it, but I didn't. Too honest, too dumb!"

"It was the right thing not to! There might be a copy elsewhere, no? Here's an idea—why don't you contact the army's health service? They might be willing to reverse their decision if you agree to give them a hand as an emergency physician in the reserve. In your position, I'd do it in order to clear my record."

"Clear my record of what? I was just a kid!"

"I know. But it could be an interesting experience for you."

"I think I should meet with the president of the General Medical Council and ask him what the fuck the original copy of my military record is doing in here!"

"You can do that, of course, but I'm not sure he'll have the answer."

~

It's curious how the notion of honor changes with age. In my youth I found it honorable to be anti-militarist. At this stage, I can choose to do nothing and let things be, even if it means that one day my past may come back at me like a boomerang when I'm least expecting it. All this strikes me as absurd, but hooked by the game and intrigued, I decide to act. I don't know it yet, but my naive curiosity is going to lead me to Afghanistan . . .

4.
PROMISED LAND

Late **November, 2008.** Three months after this episode at the
General Medical Council, I'm in Paris when I receive a strange
call on my cell phone:

"Hello, Doctor. This is the Israeli Defense Forces. I'm calling
you from Jerusalem."

It's a woman. She speaks French with no accent. Surprised and
distrustful, I ask her why she's calling.

"We're restructuring our health service," she says. "Your professional profile interests us. One of our officers is actually in
Europe for a few days. Would you be willing to meet with him?"

"How did you get my number?"

"We have our connections. You're an experienced doctor who
trained with the SAMU, a citizen of both France and Britain and
of Jewish origin, right?"

The fact is, I'm not indifferent to this phone call. I have always
been concerned about Israel and its security. Moreover, the
Israeli Defense Forces, known as Tzahal in Israel, are somewhat

mythical, and the name itself carries plenty of emotional and historical charge.

"The information you've gathered about me is correct. It's surprising because I've only been to Israel once."

"Yes, we know," she answers. "So are you willing to meet with our officer?"

All of this strikes me as bizarre. Is it really the Israeli Defense Forces? In spite of my doubts, I'm drawn by the burning bush, and I lower my guard.

"Why not?"

"He's in London. He'll call you in ten minutes to set up a meeting place."

Exactly ten minutes later, my cell rings again. I answer it. On the other end, there's a man with a serious voice. He also speaks in French, but this time with an accent I find difficult to identify.

"Hello, is this Elie?"

"Yes."

"My name is Aaron. I'm an officer with Tzahal. You already know how we operate. Can we meet tomorrow at 10 in the morning in the bar at the _____ Hotel? Near King's Cross?"

I hesitate for a moment. Then, intrigued, I agree.

During the night, I go over these phone conversations. Why me, where are these contacts coming from, did I do the right thing when I agreed to meet with them?

I start to recall my one and only trip to Israel, in 2005, during Christmas week, which coincided that year with the Jewish Festival of Lights, Hanukkah.

I was with my aging parents. It was an emotional pilgrimage for us because the experience of being in the Promised Land together was one that might never be repeated. One of my friends had put us in touch with a travel agency that specialized in the Middle East. They organized a made-to-order tour for us. An ex-commander of the Israeli Army, now retired, was our guide. His name was Shimon, and he was born in Egypt during the Second World War. His parents had emigrated to Palestine before the 1948 Arab-Israeli War. He was a solid, sixty-year-old guy who knew the hidden recesses of his country like the inside of his pocket, as he'd participated in its conflicts from the Six-Day War in 1967 through the intervention in Lebanon in 1982. Outside of his military career, he had lived in other countries and had probably worked in the secret service. He spoke French perfectly.

For a week, he led us on visits to sites that have been important in the history of three religions, and showed us some of the modern accomplishments of the young State of Israel. We got along well. Because of my dual French-British nationality and my medical experience, Shimon urged me strongly to think about collaborating professionally with his country.

"Why have you waited so many years to come to Israel, Elie?"

"Since childhood, the Promised Land has always been important to me without really attracting me."

"But you received a Jewish education?"

"Yes, but I don't go to *schul*. My family is both religious and open to other cultures."

"You're a believer?"

"I'm interested in spirituality in the larger sense of the term and in multiculturalism, but not in the orthodox side of religions. I'm allergic to dogmas presented as absolute truths; the way I see it, they only lead to fanaticism and war. Clara, my partner, is Christian. I belong to the segment of the Diaspora that's been assimilated."

"Still, you also belong to a community that's three thousand years old, one that has passed through the ordeals of all imaginable persecutions and exterminations."

"I'm aware of this, Shimon."

"Ironically, this community also gave rise to universal ideas and beings, including Jesus Christ, Spinoza, Freud, and Einstein. There aren't more than fifteen million of us in the world, but we're made responsible for all evils. . . ."

"All the more reason to get out of this vicious circle and invent other paradigms," I argued.

"That's what Israel has been trying to do since its creation," he countered, "to break the age-old image of Jews in the ghetto, constantly at the mercy of the good will and whims of the countries they live in, and to become a people that's free and proud to be so."

"I agree with you, but the problem is that Israel runs the risk of turning itself into the very ghetto we escaped! And with atomic weapons as the cherry on top!"

In answering Shimon, I was aware that he was using a kind of classic propaganda by appealing to my sense of roots, even though the content of the discussion was based on historical and contemporary realities. It's true that the State of Israel was born out of the age-old failure to integrate Jews into Europe. This anti-Judaism, then modern anti-Semitism, led to the Holocaust and the necessity of finding an asylum for the Jewish people, which was finally able to return to the land where their ancestors had lived two thousand years before.

Once that was accomplished, one might have thought that the Jewish question, as it was simplistically called, would be resolved. Instead, history went forward in a different, even more complicated manner. There's no doubt that at present, a very virulent form of contemporary anti-Semitism is growing, multiplying again under the cover of anti-Zionism, and not only in the Muslim world. A large part of international public opinion ignores the modern history of the Middle East. This fact leads to misunderstandings and hatred.

Ever since the destruction of their ancient kingdom by the

Romans, and in spite of the Diaspora, there have always been Jews remaining in Palestine. When the first Russian Jews arrived in the region, at the end of the nineteenth century, to escape the blood-thirsty pogroms, these infertile desert lands had already been legally purchased from the Ottoman Empire by Jewish bankers. The Frenchman Edmond de Rothschild, among others, had nego-tiated to pay a king's ransom for properties belonging to the Arabs. Political Zionism only developed twenty years later, in reaction to the Dreyfus affair, in the nationalist context that existed in Europe at the time.

My discussion with Shimon, in this restaurant in Jerusalem, went on. It was the first time in my life that I was in direct contact with an ex-officer of Tzahal. To top it off, I was in the Holy City. Inevitably we took up the Palestinian question from the Israeli point of view.

"Elie, Palestine comes from the Philistines, an Aegean people that settled in the area in the twelfth century BC."

"And where exactly?"

"It's unclear, but it seems to have varied depending on the period. Historically, the territory extended from the shores of the Mediterranean to the Arabian desert. In antiquity, its lands included, among others, the ancient land of Israel, the kingdom of Judah, the capital of which was Jerusalem."

"Already. . . ."

"It hadn't ever been considered a political entity by the Arabs. Four-fifths of its land was situated east of the Jordan River. Today that area forms the country of Jordan, a nation artificially cre-ated by the British after the First World War. Originally called Transjordan in 1921, it became known by its current name in 1949."

"What happened to the last fifth of the territory located to the west of the river?"

"It now covers the State of Israel, Gaza, which before 1967 was administered by Egypt, and the West Bank, which was given its name by the Transjordanians after the 1948 Arab-Israeli War."

Listening to him talk, it seems obvious that the three monotheistic religions have always cohabited on earth. Often painfully. Christianity was born here. The Arabs of the Persian Gulf came here after Prophet Muhammad's revelation in the seventh century AD. Then there were the Ottoman and British occupations. I'd read a lot on the subject and knew that in 1916, the French and British had divided up the ruins of the Ottoman Empire when they signed the Sykes-Picot Agreement without taking into account the ethno-religious identities of these populations. In other words, without those negotiations, the question of the legitimacy of all these countries, Israel included, would never even have been formulated, since none of them existed under current form at the beginning of the twentieth century. Oil has complicated the situation by playing a crucial role in all these wars for a century.

"But, Shimon, you agree there's a Palestinian problem, don't you?"

"Yes, Elie, but it's not the cause of everything, as they'd like us to believe. It has certainly been kept going by many, including the Arab countries themselves. There are those who find that ignorance and hatred suit their purposes, although the end result is always violence in both camps."

"The State of Israel could show more subtlety. Are their leaders equal to the task?"

"That's another story. There aren't any great leaders in the contemporary scene. We need a Churchill or a Gandhi to resolve this problem, which is international."

"Some have tried, however, like Anwar Sadat in Egypt and Yitzhak Rabin in Israel."

"Yes, and they were assassinated, Elie!"

~

The day after the strange phone call from Jerusalem, I go to meet with Aaron, the recruiting officer from Tzahal. It's ten o'clock in the morning. The bar in the London hotel is deserted. At the counter, waiting for me, is a man of about fifty, of average height, robust, wearing a shirt and khaki pants in colors that remind me of army clothes. He has a little black yarmulke on his bald head. He's religious, I say to myself, what does he want with a secular guy like me?

"Shalom! I'm happy to meet you, Elie," he says.

He immediately addresses me with the informal *tu*, speaking perfect French inflected with a light accent that doesn't seem Israeli in origin. His demeanor is warm, but his steel-blue eyes probe me like a laser. I learn he was born in Switzerland. His parents emigrated to Israel in the Sixties. Currently retired, he served as an officer in the Special Forces of Tzahal during the 1973 Yom Kippur War and the first war in Lebanon in 1982, receiving several special mentions for combat. As the conversation progresses, it becomes clear that I'm dealing with a radical Jew, a fact that can only turn me off.

"Okay, let's get down to business, Elie. Tzahal is an army of conscripts, and the backbone of the country. We're restructuring our health service to prepare for the eventuality of a large-scale war. It looks like your profile would suit this new organization."

"My profile?"

"We have our sources. You're a good doctor with international experience. Moreover, you're at a turning point in your life. According to the Law of Return, any Jew is eligible for Israeli citizenship. You'd be happy in Israel. . . ."

I realize as we talk that this guy who's planning my future seems to know everything about my life—that my relationship with Clara is fragile, that I have elderly parents to care for, and so forth. I have to remain calm and not allow myself to be destabilized. But finally I interrupt him.

"Who are you, the health service of the Israeli Army or the Mossad? In any case, you're wasting your breath, I can't leave Europe."

"Who's asking you to leave Europe? Our proposition is that you spend part of your time in London. In that way, you can still commute to Paris to see your family."

"Meaning?"

"You'll spend your first year in Israel. You'll learn Hebrew, then you'll familiarize yourself with the army at one of our military bases. If all goes well, you'll receive Israeli citizenship and you'll be in a position to take care of the reservists."

"Piece of cake!"

"The other part of your work will take place in England. You'll be well paid."

"What a plan! Sounds perfect!"

The officer doesn't seem to catch my irony.

At this moment of our exchange, a third man comes over to join us. A plump guy with dark hair. Unlike Aaron, he doesn't look like a fighter but more like a bureaucrat. His name is Roni, and he says he was a doctor in the Israeli Army. After a short exchange in Hebrew with his colleague, Aaron turns toward me and says, "I have to go now. I leave you with Roni. Think hard about all of this, and until soon, I hope?"

The meeting with Roni continues for two more hours. I remain guarded because I'm aware of calculation and manipulation on his part.

"Aaron spoke to you about spending two-thirds of your time in Israel and one-third in England?"

"Vaguely. . . ."

"We own a startup in medical tourism that operates out of London. The plan is for you to join our team as a medical advisor."

"Medical tourism?"

"You know the British health system well, Elie. There are things that leave a lot to be desired. . . ."

"I know, the government is in the process of reorganizing and improving it."

"Because of the history of Palestine, the Israeli medical system, just like its army, was first set up on the British model, then we adapted it to our culture and environment. At present it performs very well."

"And so?"

"We are proposing medical and surgical services of the highest quality in luxury clinics on the edge of the Mediterranean, the Red Sea, and the Dead Sea. . . ."

"Where are you going with all this?"

"We have contacts in a big British insurance agency who give us access to a list of its affiliated patients, easy to reach through a targeted information campaign. You're British and a doctor in the NHS; you could be our intermediary and inform them about our organization in Israel."

"What kinds of patients?"

"An international clientele, well-off, and of course subscribers to these private British insurance plans. You'd be paid on a commission basis. Enough to significantly increase your salary as an Israeli doctor. And then, London isn't far from Paris where you'd have the opportunity to go see your family regularly."

I observe Roni while he talks to me. With his stoutness and his slippery way of looking at me, he resembles a ball of fat that everything slides off. Nothing about him fits my idea of a Mossad agent. Nothing he tells me is sincere. It's all too good to be true. His convoluted project is surely a cover for some other one. . . .

"Does our proposition interest you?" he continues. "Are you ready to join us? If yes, we have to put things in motion straight away before you migrate to Israel."

"What do you mean by that?"

"If you give me your consent, your name will appear very soon on our startup's website. Your quick commitment would prove to us that you're motivated."

"Okay, now you're putting pressure on me. I have to think it over."

"All right. We'll be back in Europe in a month and a half. We'll meet again and you'll give us your answer. If you decide beforehand, call me. Here's my phone number in Jerusalem."

It's obvious he's trying to get me involved quickly and by any means. If I get mixed up in their system, I'll be cutting myself off from Europe without any real solution for going back, I'll lose free will, and anything could happen to me there. I could become a Mossad agent useful for other causes besides medicine, for example. The idea is seductive, appealing to my adventurous nature, and evoking a certain romantic mythology, but I'm not ready to take the leap. I still have too many ties with Europe, my family, my aging parents, my profession. I decide to test him to see his reaction.

"I have a point to add here."

"I'm listening, Elie."

"I'm actually in contact with the French Army to sort out an old dossier, and I'm being evaluated for membership in—in a certain British organization. A professional one. That agenda seems difficult, even incompatible, with your project, no?"

"Nothing is incompatible. But you'll have to make a choice. Stay in Europe or emigrate to Israel. Go ahead, become a member of whatever organization you want. It's all good for us. Your contact with the French Army isn't an obstacle if you straighten out your situation. But if you join up with us, you'll be Israeli and a member of Tzahal. Let me repeat, you have to make a choice!"

I leave very troubled by this conversation, still not understanding either the scope of the project, which seems legally dubious, or why I've been targeted. In any case, he doesn't seem ready to spill the beans. It all seems like a trap, a manipulation. Are these two guys really recruiters for Tzahal, representing a constructive project, or are they Mossad agents? Maybe they're both at the same time! Or simply crooks out for their own gain . . . I'd better be careful.

5.
THE FRENCH ARMY

End of 2008. It'll be Christmas soon. In London, my work is going full steam ahead. Concerned by what happened at the General Medical Council, I have finally resolved to go back to Paris and meet with the French Army in order to straighten out my military record.

Rémi, a veteran of the Special Forces, has gotten me an appointment for early January. He and I have been very close ever since I helped his youngest brother quit hard drugs. I have faith in him. He's an honest guy who has risked his life several times for his country, France. When I talked to him about my military past, he spontaneously proposed to help me. Regarding the Israelis, his reaction was immediate. "The Mossad! I completed a few intelligence missions in Lebanon and know a bit about their methods. The startup and medical tourism projects are probably a cover. If you join them, it'll be difficult for you to keep your ties with France and the United Kingdom."

"If that's the case, what should I do?"

"You should break off all contact. All the more so because you've asked the French Army to straighten out your situation. You don't have any choice, you have to speak to the French, because if they learn about it through some other source, you run the risk of being taken for an Israeli agent. Those guys have put you in a tight corner."

"I'm supposed to see them again in a month and a half."

"The French Army colonel you're going to meet with soon— you can ask him for advice about what to do."

The sequence of events is obviously strange to me. If Rémi is right, I've gotten myself into a real fix! I should have ignored my military dossier and never responded to the advances made to me by those so-called Israelis. I have the feeling that, in acting as I did, I tempted fate.

~

Early January 2009. Ten o'clock in the morning. I've arrived from London on the first Eurostar of the day. For me, this date is memorable because I haven't set foot in the army since I got myself thrown out over thirty years ago. What a strange impression the scene makes on me, this military camp covered in snow on a beautiful winter's morning. The grounds are landscaped. It feels bizarre to be here again.

Elie, my grandfather, walks by my side. The deeper I sink into this story, the more he appears to me. I imagine him in the uniform of the second Algerian regiment of *Zouaves*, the troops from the French territories in North Africa. I see him right before an attack. He's freezing in the trenches, there's both fear in his belly and a stubborn faith in his own survival, he's got a helmet on his head, a dirty, worn uniform on his back, and a bayonet in his hand. A last gulp of hard stuff before hearing the "Forward!" command yelled out by an officer ready to shoot down those men who won't advance into the enemy's murderous fire.

Truth is, my grandfather didn't even drink the alcohol they gave him. My father told me he exchanged it for cigarettes. Either he was damned lucky to get out of there alive, or he had guardian angels. He'd think I was nuts to be here today.

For the time being, here I am seated, waiting for my appointment with a colonel who is supposed to straighten out my military dossier and resolve the so-called mistakes of my youth. Surreal!

"The chief physician is expecting you," says a secretary in uniform. "Fourth office on the right."

I make my way across the beige waxed parquet of a long, impersonal hall with white walls, looking for my interlocutor. The door to his office is open. A rather elegant man in military uniform comes toward me. His manner is cold, but that's only my first impression.

"Hello!" I say. "Should I address you as 'Doctor'?"

"Call me Chief Physician or Colonel. I see you're not familiar with the institution."

"That's right, I didn't serve in the army."

"Unusual for a doctor, no?"

"I wasn't a doctor when it happened. I was twenty and a musician. I studied medicine later on."

"They declared you unfit?"

"Let's say I did everything possible to make it happen—really stupid things!"

"Everyone did. Why are you contacting us after all this time?"

"I wouldn't have approached you if I hadn't accidentally stumbled across the original copy of my military dossier."

"Meaning?"

"I don't know why, but it turns out that it's in my professional dossier at the General Medical Council."

"I agree with you, it should have been archived. But after all, what does it matter, there's a statute of limitations."

"Maybe! But if it's in my civilian dossier, I'm no longer protected by military secrecy. It's a mess that could come out at any time. I don't like this idea. Especially because the report was really spiced up and doesn't reflect my true personality. I overplayed things to get myself thrown out. The psychiatrist understood this and went along with it, that's all."

"Whether or not it reflects reality, the report exists, and we can only retrieve it if you come back to the army."

"By which you mean what exactly, Colonel?"

"We have to reevaluate you psychologically, physically, and militarily. For that to happen, you'll have to go before military doctors and psychiatrists once more; then, if you're declared fit, we'll integrate you into the reserve."

"And what would that involve?"

"For a doctor, doing a minimum of one five-day stint a year in the army health service."

"Nothing more?"

"Your case is a little different. You're in a tough spot here. You have a problematic history with us. Moreover, your CV is atypical and interesting. International physician, athletic, and still in good shape. A perfect profile for serving in the active reserve and giving us a helping hand—in Afghanistan, for example!"

"That's all? To take care of an old problem that shouldn't have existed in the first place? Frankly, it's not my fault if my military dossier turned up in my civilian one. Many young people of my generation found a way out of serving in the army. Besides, today military service is no longer required."

"I know, but you're a physician from the last generation. There's no getting around that fact!"

"But you'll admit that it's pretty wild. I reappear thirty years later, and you suggest I go to Afghanistan! Are you short of volunteers in the army? I'd rather do nothing, and leave my military dossier right where it never should have been!"

"Think it over! Maybe it won't be Afghanistan. Everything will depend on what our strategy is at the time. On the other hand, we are in need of emergency physicians in our military hospitals right outside Paris. You could do a few shifts there, even if you're still based in the UK. That would probably be enough for you to sort out your dossier. What do you think?"

"That seems like an acceptable proposition."

"In any case, it'll take some time before everything gets resolved. I'd like to propose that we meet again in the spring. Between now and then, you will have perhaps reached a decision. Don't wait too long."

"Why?"

"After summer, it'll be harder to set the process in motion. The army is a ponderous institution. We organize our schedules and reach decisions several months in advance. And I might no longer be here to follow up on the matter. Take advantage of this opportunity."

"I hear you! I have one last thing to tell you before I leave. I'm not sure it's the right thing to do, but a friend of mine in the military strongly urged me to talk to you about it."

"What's this about?"

"Listen, I was recently approached by officers from the Israeli Army."

"And you met with them?"

"Yes, in London."

"What did they want?"

"They proposed that I should emigrate to Israel and work as a physician in the Tzahal Reserve."

"That makes sense, you're Jewish and they're interested in you."

"That's not all. They'd like me to spend one third of my time in the United Kingdom to work with an Israeli startup that does medical tourism."

"The Mossad!"

"You think so?"

"Yes, that's how they operate! They recruit you for a particular reason, then make you do something else. They're trying to drag you into who knows what! You never should have met with them."

"I didn't know . . . They played on my feelings—Judaism, Zionism, my ancestors. . . ."

"They knew what they were doing when they appealed to your sentimentality about your roots! If you accept, there'll be no going back. With them on your back, you'll be in a delicate situation on French territory. They know that. They'll stick the Secret Services up your ass. And then—hello!—you'll be blacklisted indefinitely!"

"You're trying to manipulate me!"

"Not really! For the moment, let's keep this business between you and me. It's yet another reason for you to think long and hard before making a decision and joining us in the reserve."

"Meaning?"

"The fact of joining the reserve will protect you. You're standing at the intersection of three countries—France, the UK, and Israel. The British Services maybe already know that the Israelis approached you. Be very careful. You're going to have to make a choice, and the right one."

"On top of everything else, I have informal and friendly contacts with people in the Foreign Office. And I'm undergoing a professional evaluation at the Royal College of Physicians."

"You see! The British are tracking you, too! Who were these people at the Foreign Office?"

"A couple I met at some friends', in London. We hit it off, and saw each other a few more times. They've been posted to different British embassies throughout the world."

"Maybe a coincidence, or maybe not. You have to stay on your guard!"

"I wonder why all these people are so interested in me."

"That's how it is, your profile resonates with current needs. And you would seem to be the right man for what's ahead."

"What do you advise me to do?"

"You're French and British. Your family is in Europe. If you choose Israel, you'll be cutting yourself off from them. It'll be difficult for you to come back. Stop all contact with the Israeli Services!"

"I already have a meeting with them set up for a couple of weeks from now."

"Okay, go to it, and tell them you're declining their offer. Mention your ties with us. There's still time."

"I'll be obliged to return to France if I serve in the reserve?"

"Not necessarily. As I said, you can come do your periods of duty and your shifts while remaining based in London. You can approach it as a return to the origins of your work at the SAMU. After all, the French emergency services, which you know well, were established on the military model of frontline medicine. Keep me up to date immediately as things develop. Good luck!"

As I leave the military camp, the situation seems even more complex than it had before. I hadn't seen any of it coming, and I've gotten myself into a real pickle. A sucker taken in by a gang of con artists, caught behind the eight ball.

6.

MARINE COMMANDOS

Spring 2010. Here I am, dear reader, sending you greetings from Lorient in Brittany, where I am in training on the base of FORFUSCO, the home of the Marine Commandos. I'm a captain in the operational reserve of the French Army Health Service. Given my history, it's rather ironic.

The preceding year, shortly after my last encounter with the Israelis, the pace of events accelerated. Following the recommendation of the French physician colonel, I scheduled a meeting with them in order to decline their offer. It was a tough encounter.

Aaron and Roni were joined by a woman this time.

"What have you decided?" Aaron asked.

"What do you mean? Are you brothers or enemies? You got me into deep shit," I said. "The French military is now suspicious of me. And you knew this would happen when you contacted me."

The woman intervened. "A Jew doesn't talk like you."

"What? 'A Jew doesn't talk like me'? The Jews have been around for three thousand years, the Diaspora for two thousand,

and the State of Israel for a mere sixty-five! No way—you can't hijack my identity!"

"But we in Israel," Roni said, "are fighting for the Jewish people. You in Europe are doing nothing for us."

"How can you say such a thing? My grandfather Elie fought in the shit-filled trenches at Verdun for four years. And my father's generation fought during World War II so you could exist afterwards. How can you compare that to the Six-Day War?"

As we spoke, I became aware of my two clashing identities— the first as a European, the second as a Sephardic Jew.

"If that's your attitude, okay. We liked you but you've made your choice."

Rightly or wrongly, I felt that they wouldn't let me go that easily. Who were they? I wanted to find out the truth. Believing I was solving the problem, I contacted the Israeli embassy in London. Just the thing not to do, because everyone, except me at the time, knows that embassies the world over are spy dens. It only complicated the matter. Evidently, no one knew anything about it, and they sent me back home.

A little later, I received a letter from the Royal College of Physicians, announcing, with the cold politeness of the English, that I would never be a member of their venerable institution. *No comment.* The doors were closed on me. Why this reversal? Was it connected to the Foreign Office or the Israelis? I have no idea.

My path in the United Kingdom suddenly seemed blocked. Isolated, I thought then that it would be best for me to leave London and go back to living in Paris with my family. From there it would be an easy step to join the French Army. Several factors led me to take their offer seriously. First, the army implicitly offered me protection and normalization of my military dossier. And then it provided me with work, because returning to one's country after ten years of absence isn't an easy thing. A job as an emergency physician in a military hospital was thus welcome. Finally, if they sent me abroad, the upside was that work outside France was remunerated at twice the normal salary. Reasons that seemed practical, far from any kind of patriotic feeling.

That wasn't the whole story, for, essentially, I'm not materialistic. I had more idealistic motives, which, as I saw it, made sense. The fight against jihadism, this new fascism, for example. Not having responded to the advances of the Israelis, I had deep inside me a sense of having left something unfinished, as though I hadn't sworn allegiance to the common history of the Jewish people. I know this feeling came out of the narrative I'd made about my relationship to Judaism, but it bothered me nonetheless. Joining the French Army, an ally of the Americans—the principal supporters of the Israelis widely implicated in the global war against terrorism—relieved me of my guilt. I thought about my grandfather constantly. A tangible way of reconnecting with my ancestral routes in order not to drown in troubled waters. Permanent and soothing, this internal presence seemed to push me in that direction.

These rather naive motives helped me, at the time, to make difficult choices and go through a trial by fire. You do what you can, there's nothing ridiculous about wanting to survive. Today, after having lived in Afghanistan and experienced the reality of its terrain, I understand a little better the complexity of these conflicts in which religious ideology has become central, and I reflect about it differently.

I could have said no to the army and refused to sign up. But circumstances were such that I found myself stuck, a cog in a machine with no exit. It then became more complicated to refuse than to accept. I could no longer back out. At the end of the day, the adventure wouldn't displease me. I must be one of those beings who are enlivened by risks and adrenalin, when they aren't destroyed by them. In Afghanistan, coming into contact with the fighters, I learned the two qualities essential for a soldier: the sense of ultimate sacrifice that is the gift of one's life, and luck, because one needs it in order to come back whole. A hard but fruitful experience.

~

Return to the FORFUSCO base. It's eight o'clock in the morning. Standing to attention in my uniform with a beret on my head, I witness the daily parade. I belong to a group of health professionals. Nurses, veterinarians and doctors, we're there to familiarize ourselves with military life.

The training focuses on discipline, sports, and the handling of weapons. The camp is spread out and located on the edge of the sea. The Marine Commandos, being the marine component of the French Army's Special Forces, train hard here for battle, on land and sea. Parachuting, swimming, diving, climbing, combat sports, firearms, knives are all included. Psychological pressure is constant, and the strengthening of mental qualities is essential. Their doctors are also highly trained.

I know that all of this is just an initiation, a test to measure our psychological and physical qualities, as well as our ability to adapt ourselves to the group and the rules of military life. Those in the reserve are rarely deployed to war zones. My friend Rémi, a veteran of the Special Forces, has warned me, "You can't learn to be a soldier so fast. This is only a beginning."

When I decided to join the reserve, after the medical visit, I was declared healthy in mind and body and ready to be operational. Which means that at any time I might have to leave on "OPEX", or "external operations." To stay ahead of the game, Rémi, sensing what would happen to me, taught me how to shoot at his club. We went there every week and together worked with handguns—SIG, Glock, HK—as well as assault weapons such as the French FAMAS, the American M16, the German HK, and the Russian Kalashnikov AK-47.

At the same time, I took my physical condition in hand again. An old buddy, a former professional boxer in the English style, coached me at the boxing club he runs in Paris. As in the good old days, I found myself training twice a week with the jumping rope, the punching bag, and doing shadowboxing or sparring with him, so as to work on technique and reflexes. In order to complete everything, I did forty-five minutes of jogging, three times a week, and some indoor rock climbing.

Although I was in my fifties, I didn't find it difficult to make a comeback because, ever since my days of university boxing, I had never completely stopped doing sports. I've focused on mountain climbing, diving, and yoga, the sport of sports.

"Normally a military doctor is not supposed to train like a fighter, except if they are attached to the commandos. But you, Elie, they stuck in the operational reserve."

"Which means what, Rémi?"

"That they can send you to a theater of operations in Afghanistan, for example."

"The colonel who recruited me told me that wouldn't happen."

"With the army, a no can easily turn into a yes, and vice-versa. It's a question of circumstance and opportunity. Don't forget that you signed up for five years. They're watching you."

"If that's the case, I'm in real trouble."

"Trust me, I know from experience, you need to continue to do your own training because they're not going to do it for you. They have neither the time nor the money. They know your physical and mental potential, they recruited you for that, so show them you're self-sufficient, the way you always have. That's what they're expecting of you."

I followed Rémi's advice until my departure for Afghanistan eighteen months later. I'm glad I did so because this trip across the new continent that the army was for me turned out to be complicated and full of traps all the way through.

Contrary to expectations, my acculturation with the Marine Commandos turned out to be rich and fruitful. I liked the competence, the courage, and commitment of these elite units of the French Navy. I got along well with these tough, top-level guys, whom I would meet up with again at Djibouti, an obligatory stop on the way to Afghanistan.

Consisting of six units, the Marine Commandos were created during World War II. The oldest one, the Kieffer Commando, was founded in 1942 by the British intelligence service. Trained in Scotland, these men fought in the Free French Forces. They have been in difficult places, both on land and sea, and have performed exceptional missions in Indochina, Algeria, Africa, Afghanistan, and elsewhere. Today they still wear the green beret they earned at the time of their creation, a mythical symbol of the British Special Forces. An onsite museum traces their history and that of the French Navy from the first royal troops created by Cardinal Richelieu, the prime minister of Louis XIV, until today.

While visiting the museum, I stop before a headquarters map, dating from the Algerian War, of Nemours, the fishing port where I was born. Astonished, I turn to the ex-commando who is acting as my guide. "This is unbelievable, I was born in this building, where my parents lived with my grandparents, on this very avenue facing the sea! For strategic reasons, the French Navy requisitioned it."

"What a coincidence, Doc!"

"Before leaving Algeria, my grandfather started a procedure to get it back. This went on for three years, and he died while it was in process. The navy finally indemnified my family for the move, but not very much."

"It was wartime. . . ."

"That's besides the point. On the other hand, we would have had to leave Algeria sooner or later, anyway. History proved us right; moreover, one of my uncles had been drafted into that war, and my father would be called up for the territorial army. It was getting to be too much."

"I'm moved by what you're telling me, Doc. At present, you're with us. It's a fair turn of events, a kind of resilience?"

"Fair, I'm not sure about that. But in fact it's disturbing. It's as though a long cycle that began with my birth is coming to completion."

"Another cycle is about to begin."

Decidedly, the recurrence shaped my trajectory. I had to integrate myself into the Marine Commandos in order to come face to face with my paternal family. Even if there was some kind of manipulation in what had been happening to me for two years, it couldn't have gone that far. Only the hand of destiny could partly explain what was going on, as though I had to do some compensatory work for my family in order to reestablish a harmony that would have been broken, for what reasons I don't know. All this struck me as strange.

~

A week after my return from Lorient, I received a phone call from an officer from headquarters.

"Given your aptitudes and the quality of your performance, we've decided to deploy you to Djibouti this summer. You'll be posted as an emergency doctor, which will give you an opportunity to become familiar with the Marine Commandos and the French Foreign Legion. Among other things, they're doing intensive training for Afghanistan. We're also trying out our equipment. Are you satisfied?"

"Do I have a choice?"

"You can always say no, but don't forget you have a deal with us. And then you'll get to have experiences. Between now and your departure, I advise you to continue working on your physical condition and to practice shooting. Congratulations!"

I remained doubtful. What was supposed to be simple emergency shifts in a Parisian military hospital has taken a strange turn. I would later understand that when the army entrusts you with a mission, it's an honor.

7.
DJIBOUTI

Summer 2010. Arrival in the Horn of Africa. Six o'clock in the
morning. The sun is already intense and the heat humid. The
unique odor hanging thick in the air is strong and vegetal, like that
of damp compost. I've changed continents in the space of a single
night and it's obvious. The civilian airplane I traveled in from
Paris is full of Djiboutians as well as French and American military personnel. The airport, surrounded by the desert, seems to be
in the middle of nowhere. At the entrance to customs, I observe
rainbow-colored frescoes in a naive style and a panel with words
written in French, English and Arabic: "Welcome to Djibouti."

A crowd dressed in colorful clothing lines up in the envelop-
ing din. Djiboutian soldiers are everywhere. The customs inspec-
tion lasts a long time. Recovering our baggage takes forever. It's
another world where everything seems disorganized.

Finally, a French sergeant locates me in the middle of this
chaos. Soon we're driving toward the Bouffard French Military
Hospital, located near the center of the capital, which, like the

country itself, is called Djibouti. The van is air-conditioned. What a contrast with the heat outside!

"Welcome to the Horn of Africa, Captain!" Even as he drives, he notices my interest and astonishment as I discover this new environment. Djibouti is one of the smallest states of the continent, covering an area about one sixth of England.

The road to the hospital is in bad condition. It's a desert landscape. We cross through several inhabited zones that are clearly very poor. The houses are dilapidated.

"You'll see, East Africa is very special and engaging," the sergeant says. "It'll soon be two years that I've been posted here. I'd stay longer if I could." He goes on to talk about the warmth of the people and the beauty of this volcanic, magnetic landscape lying on the great fault between Africa and Asia.

The periodic appearance of mosques reminds me that I'm in a Muslim country. The population consists of an astonishing mixture of people from Africa and the Middle East.

Skin color is dark brown veering toward black, facial traits are delicate. Women, often veiled, wear brightly colored clothes. White, turquoise blue, orange, and pink appear even more intense in this African light, already very strong in the early morning. A part of the population seems to live outside. Goats roam freely in the streets. Dust hangs everywhere, inescapable. My first impression is one of misery exposed under the sun.

"People are very poor here, Sergeant?"

"Yes. Whole families live in cardboard boxes rigged up as houses, they wash and do their business in the Red Sea. And then there's khat!"

"I've heard about it," I say. Khat is a psychoactive plant that grows in Ethiopia and Yemen.

"It's one of the scourges of this country and the Horn of Africa. It's the national drug. Everybody consumes it here, from the president and his wife, who seem to hold a monopoly on its trafficking, to the most poverty-stricken, including the army and police in between. As for women, they consume it secretly. Huge quantities of khat arrive in Djibouti every morning, and people rush to the port to buy some. It's best not to be out and about at that time of day."

"I didn't realize it was such a widespread phenomenon."

"You'll see, Doc, that addicts chew it for hours, keeping in their mouths balls of it you can easily spot because their cheeks are puffed up with the stuff. They call that 'grazing.'"

"At that rate, they don't have a chance of escaping poverty. Without getting cynical about it, one can wonder whether, on top of bringing in money, the khat trade isn't also a way of controlling the population. People can't engage in revolution when they're slumped over half the time, stoned from chewing their drug of choice."

Grazing produces a bitter juice that makes people very thirsty, with the consequence that users tend to drink quarts of locally manufactured, overly sweetened Coca-Cola. Secondary effects don't take long to appear. They can be devastating and include cardiovascular illnesses, diabetes, and behavioral disorders. In this place, people don't grow old.

"Who runs the country, Sergeant?"

"Djibouti is officially a Muslim republic. However, it's governed by a dictator."

"Another banana republic, controlled by Western powers?"

"That's for sure, this little country has its own revolving doors. We French have been based here since the end of the nineteenth century."

"Arthur Rimbaud traveled in the region around the same time and wrote about it in his letters," I say, mentioning one of my favorite French poets, whose correspondence I've read with fascination.

"I know, and I've heard that Rimbaud advised the emperor of Abyssinia, Menelik, and might also have helped the French military to settle in the region."

"The country has a strategic position?" I ask.

"Yes, at the crossroads between the Orient and the West, on the maritime axes of Europe, the Far East, the Persian Gulf and, obviously, Africa. Because it's located at a commercial and military crossroads, Djibouti has been coveted by many. "

"I'm beginning to understand better why not only the French but also the Americans are interested in it."

"Not only the Americans, Captain. The Japanese, Arabs, and Chinese too. For Americans, this country has become a major fulcrum. In 2002, they established their military base at Camp Lemonier in order to control terrorist activities in the Gulf region and pirates on the Indian Ocean."

"What about Arab countries and the Chinese? Do they also have a presence here?"

"The Arabs see here opportunities that are above all economic and ideological. Saudi Arabia is investing a lot of money in religious propaganda and building brand-new mosques with gold roofs. As for the Chinese, they're establishing themselves everywhere in Africa."

"The Chinese-American battle for hegemony."

"So to speak! You may also hear people speak about slavery, Doc."

"Really? But slavery is most often associated with America, the English, and the French, and more generally with the white man."

"People forget to mention that it's an economic system going back to antiquity, and that the Arabs have never stopped practicing it. The black man isn't a stranger to it either, for he has also profited from the slave trade by selling his own brothers. Djibouti has for centuries been a transit zone for African slaves sold in the Middle East."

He knows what he's talking about. Indeed, later during my stay in Djibouti, I was traveling on the road to the port of Tadjoura on the edge of the Red Sea, where I would see men and women marching in the desert, people who, hoping for jobs, have been deceived into leaving their country. Chosen by their tribal chiefs, they take boats from Obok on the edge of the Red Sea for Yemen; they are headed for Saudi Arabia, where they will enter modern slavery. I wasn't even allowed to give them water.

As I watch the landscape go by, I imagine Arthur Rimbaud getting off a ship here, at the time it was being colonized by the French. The climate must have been as hot as it is today, and life even more dangerous. How did this genius of a poet end up in this land, far from the civilization of which he would, one day, be considered a jewel? Almost ignored by his era, he didn't know he would influence the surrealist poets, the Americans and the Beat Generation, including Jack Kerouac, and then Bob Dylan. He was not only an arms trader, he also drew maps of the area, discovered new trade routes, was a great horseman, and became a student of the area's languages. In short, he was an explorer. His adventurous spirit has inspired me since I first read his poems as a teenager.

Our conversation is interrupted when we reach Bouffard military hospital. The building, in the colonial style, is located along the old train tracks connecting Djibouti with Ethiopia. This line used to be ridden by the sovereign, or negus, of Ethiopia, Haile Selassie. Today it is barely used. A train passes this way only from time to time.

Bouffard is a small structure providing all basic services including emergency care, resuscitation, a surgical department, radiology, a laboratory, and a pharmacy. It is surrounded by white walls along which you can see sitting, 24/7, poor, passive, and idle men completely anesthetized and destroyed by khat. They seem reassured by the presence of the hospital, although they never have access to care there. For the hospital serves exclusively the French, American, and allied military, the local army and police, and the country's high-ranking civil servants and VIPs, as well as the families of all these people. No time or space for the truly down-and-out, and no exceptions!

There I meet Bertrand, my colleague and roommate, a physician reservist who has come to reinforce the internal medicine department. A robust guy of sixty-two from Alsace, likable and open. Our relationship is very friendly from the start. We visit the different sites together, an occasion to meet the teams I've been called upon to work with.

Bertrand will later tell me that during the Soviet–Afghan War, he served in the French Army's intelligence service in Afghanistan, under the cover of an NGO. At the time of the Cold War, the Americans, British, and French had supported the Afghan *mujahideen* against the Soviets. Bertrand has known this country and its mysteries since the 1970s. He was at that time, and still is, a preeminent cavalryman. Back then, he traveled far and wide and on horseback. He understood the languages and mentality of the different ethnicities constituting this fascinating land. During his missions, he'd met the famous Ahmad Shah Massoud, the military commander who led the resistance against the Soviet occupation and was assassinated on September 9, 2001, two days before the attack on the Twin Towers in New York. A man who had resisted the Taliban and been open to the West and to France, especially.

I would realize later that Bertrand had been assigned to me as a roommate for a reason: to track and observe my adaptive abilities as I made my way to Afghanistan.

∾

At Bouffard, we also take care of the health of the Marine Commandos, the Foreign Legion, and the Air Commandos. Everyone is trained at Djibouti before being deployed wherever France needs them to go. The predominant destination is, at this moment in 2010, Afghanistan. Later on, the Foreign Legion will leave the site in order to base itself in Abu Dhabi before returning to France.

There's a wide spectrum of departments, including pediatrics, obstetrics–gynecology, infectious and tropical diseases, visceral surgery, orthopedics, neurosurgery, otolaryngology, and ophthalmology. From time to time, wounded patients arrive from Somalia or from the fight against sea pirating, as well as from the American military. As the US Army hospital isn't, as of 2010, completely functional, we take care of their emergencies. I've learned that in this context, in war zones, medicine cannot be separated from politics and diplomacy.

Camp Lemonier, originally used by the French Foreign Legion, is now a huge, five-star US Navy complex, built in a deserted zone of the city, with a pool, movie theaters, gym rooms, restaurants, supermarkets, internet, and high-tech equipment within easy reach, all provided with typical American knowhow. My father often said to me, "When the Yankees go to war, they move around as comfortably as possible, with their own food and water." I've learned through personal experience that this is true. Their logistics at Djibouti are gigantic.

The USA remains, for the moment, the foremost world power. A real war machine. Massive amounts of money are invested in this business. Following the Roman model, they know that they have to make war in order for their *Pax Americana* to rule. The infantry enjoy a level of comfort that is much superior to the French and British. A superior officer in the French Army once threw out the following comment, joking, "On the ground, with the American soldier, it's almost as though someone's going to carry his assault weapon and backpack for him, or a helicopter's going to resupply him when he's hungry."

During my visit to the camp, I reflect that an excess of comfort can lead to less autonomy. French and British infantrymen have lesser means but know how to handle hardship. When there are hard knocks, they are prepared because they have been trained to live with the minimum.

As already suggested, Djibouti is a revolving door. Its luxurious palace, decorated in a flamboyant oriental style and situated on the edge of the Red Sea, is a meeting place for international business and intelligence services. Businessmen and traffickers of all kinds rub elbows here, in a hush-hush, shady atmosphere.

Jeff belongs to this top-level network. He is a mysterious and colorful character, maybe one of the most influential men in the Horn of Africa. A friend of his, a French officer, introduced me to him. Born in Ethiopia and an Orthodox Christian like the majority of Ethiopians, Jeff is a fervent believer. His mother came from Haile Selassie's family. His father was of Indian origin. This combination has given him a very distinctive appearance. Always smiling, of average height, thin and elegant, he has fair skin while his facial features have the refinement of Ethiopians combined subtly with the features of inhabitants of the Indian continent.

In the Cold War era, the Negus Haile Selassie was rather inclined toward the Western camp. When he was deposed and then assassinated by opponents tied to the communist regimes, Jeff's family fled and settled in Djibouti, under the protection of the French Army. I understood the complexity of his character and his indestructible warmth for France when, after we'd met several times, he told me his life story.

In Djibouti, he's officially in the import-export business— apparently, because when you have the privilege of being invited to his office, you suddenly penetrate into another universe. He receives you like royalty. French wines and champagnes of the best vintages, superb dishes from the Horn of Africa and the Middle East are all served with class by his maître d'. The whole gives you the singular and subtle impression of African, oriental, and French hospitality mixed and infused with British composure.

His office is rather large and furnished in the English style, its atmosphere both warm and baroque, with red and green predominating. Photos featuring Jeff with important world figures cover the walls. Here he is smiling next to Pope John Paul II, there he is as a child with the Negus Haile Selassie, Emperor of Ethiopia, and in yet other pictures he can be seen with different presidents of the French Republic. To the left of his armchair, there's a statue of the Virgin Mary that's about one and a half meters high. He has a real devotion to her, though I never find out why.

All kinds of influential people pass through his place—officers from the French Army, businessmen, and other mysterious people. Given his connections in the Horn of Africa and the Middle East, Jeff must undoubtedly function as an interface between France and its allies, at the intersection of intelligence, diplomacy, and business. When I ask him how he manages to export shipments of alcohol to countries on the Arabian Peninsula, where it is prohibited, he answers mischievously, "Oh, you know, Elie, over there they drink whiskey out of teacups!"

I won't see Jeff again, but this meeting makes me aware of the complex and opaque nature of international relations. A good initiation into the shadow world on my way to Afghanistan.

As I leave Djibouti, my mind wanders back to the poet Rimbaud, whose youthful rebelliousness I can identify with. And I'm aware that my trajectory has certain points in common with his. Just as my family served in the military and had lived in Algeria, so Rimbaud's father was an infantry captain who'd participated in the conquest of Algeria in the mid-nineteenth century. Still a rebellious adolescent after his break with his lover, the poet Verlaine, he stopped writing and joined the Dutch Legion, only to desert it a few months later. An adventurer, he was in his early twenties and had already traveled in many parts of the world before he arrived in the Horn of Africa. Was he, consciously or unconsciously, retracing the steps of his father, Captain Rimbaud? That's the question I ask myself as I remember the poem in prose he wrote right before leaving for Africa, later published in *Une saison en enfer* (1873):

> *I wait for God greedily. I belong to an inferior race for all eternity.*
>
> *Here I am on the beach of Brittany. May the cities be lit up in the evening. My day is done; I'm leaving Europe. Sea air will burn my lungs; lost climates will tan my skin. To swim, crush the grass, hunt, above all smoke; to drink liquors as strong as boiling metal, the way our dear ancestors did around their fires.*
>
> *I will return, with limbs of iron, dark skin, a furious eye: from my mask, they will conclude I'm from a strong race. I will have gold: I will be idle and brutal. Women take care of these ferocious invalids, back from the hot countries. I will be drawn into political affairs. Saved.*
>
> *(Trans. J.L.)*

As I stand on the threshold to Afghanistan, Rimbaud is my mentor and my inspiration, for, like him, I am experiencing, stronger than fear or anxiety, the elation that comes at the beginning of an adventure that will test one's capacities to the utmost. In spite of my adversity to war, I am also attracted by it as a trial, an initiation into the warrior archetype. In the horrible scenes that await me, I will, like this poet, go through some kind of alchemical transformation. If I survive and return unharmed, I hope I will be a stronger, more self-reliant and generous human being.

8.
YORK

Summer 2011. I'm traveling to Afghanistan. Almost three hours that we've been traveling in this military airplane, destination Dushanbe in Tajikistan.

Deep in reflection, I'm not aware of the passage of time. The atmosphere is silent. Some of the soldiers are sleeping. Others read or, like me, are absorbed in their thoughts. While daydreaming, I can follow the progress of the flight on the screen hooked onto the back of the seat in front of me. Before long, the flight captain announces our scheduled stop in Cyprus.

The layover lasts three hours. It's an opportunity to have a coffee and eat something at the airport bar. Tired, I stretch out on a bench at some distance from the others and fall asleep.

Suddenly I'm awakened by a voice on the loudspeaker announcing that we're about to leave again. Too bad, because I was in the middle of a dream. It's six thirty in the morning. I must have slept two hours. Back on the airplane, I watch *The Cincinnati Kid* on my laptop. Steve McQueen and Edward G. Robinson. Guys with class!

They serve us a meal toward noon. The screen shows that at the present moment, we are flying over Israel in the direction of the Gulf States. I pick up my book about Afghanistan again. I'm finding it hard to concentrate.

Little by little, I sink back into the movie of my own life, and my thoughts tumble along in a rush.

I see myself at the age of twenty-six again, sitting in a movie theater in the Latin Quarter, watching *Meetings with Remarkable Men*, a full-length film directed by Peter Brook. Then deciding, right after the screening, to go to medical school.

Filmed entirely in Afghanistan right before the Soviet–Afghan War of 1979, this meditative and metaphysical film retraces the adventurous life of the young George Gurdjieff, traveling through the magnificent landscapes of Central Asia at the end of the nineteenth century, during the war between the Russians and the British. Thirsty for spirituality, he was seeking secret and initiatory brotherhoods. Often disparaged, the Armenian Gurdjieff was an adventurer fascinated by esoteric subjects and would have a considerable influence in the twentieth century on those segments of European and American elites interested in Orientalism and Theosophy, then in vogue. Afghanistan would be a key step in his initiatory journey.

When I stepped into that movie theater, I hadn't yet heard of Gurdjieff, but the story of his quest for meaning, at the opposite extreme of my superficial life as a musician, resonated with me, striking a sensitive cord that set me in motion. I was attracted to the mystical ambiance of the film, and it made me think about the big picture of my life, about how I might align my work with my values and with spiritual principles. The only way I could find to do that was through medicine. In fact, I'd been waiting for a trigger of this kind for a long time, and it happened that day, at the right moment. Suddenly I was sure of it—I wanted to live the kind of life he'd led, full of adventure and humanity, focused on serving others. I was ready to exchange my musician's garb for that of a medical student.

Years later, after I'd become a doctor, I ended up, by a curious coincidence, living in the London building where Ouspenski, Gurdjieff's alter ego and traveling companion, had once lived. It so happens that between the two wars, Piotr Demianovitch Ouspenski, the Russian philosopher and mathematician, had spread Gurdjieff's metaphysical thinking as well as his own ideas in the high spheres of the British intelligentsia.

Astonishingly, as I was moving into my new apartment, the manager of the building asked me if I'd seen *Meetings with Remarkable Men*. Amazed by his question, I answered that the film had influenced the course of my life. He then informed me that Peter Brook and his main actor, Terence Stamp, had stayed in that house during the movie's production.

Even more disturbing and mysterious, here I am now a military doctor on my way to Afghanistan, apparently not for the same reasons as Gurdjieff, unless this journey is meant to be initiatory for me as well. I'd then be coming full circle.

This country in Central Asia has thus been in my life since the spring afternoon in my past, long ago, that I spent in a movie theater in the Latin Quarter, the Cluny Palace, which has long since closed. In an ironic twist of fate, right before my departure, I bought a map of Afghanistan in a travel bookstore on the Boulevard Saint-Germain, a few steps from the old cinema. Recurrence or synchronicity, I don't know, but I'm suddenly, on the airplane, overcome by a bizarre feeling of déjà-vu.

$\sim$

Shortly before my Afghan mission, the French Army finally fulfilled its promise and contacted the General Medical Council in

Paris. I was thus able to recuperate the military dossier from my youth. The president of the council received me. "The whole time I've worked in this institution, I've never seen anything like this. Your case is truly bizarre! The armies' health service sent me an official letter asking me to put your old military dossier directly in your hands. If I understand correctly from what they've told me in their letter, you're at present a captain in the operational reserve?"

"That's correct, I've already served in Djibouti, and I'm getting ready to leave for Afghanistan. In any case, there was no reason for my military dossier to end up with you. It's illegal."

"You're doing all this to take care of this miserable dossier?"

"Miserable for you, but not for me. It has become a professional liability. "

"It will be handed over to you at an official meeting, with a lawyer from the council and myself present."

This whole adventure remains incomprehensible to me, even Kafkaesque. What role is free will playing in this story, and what role destiny? Certain circumstances are apparently given. Does one, as the mystics suggest, really choose the family one is born into, the manner of one's death, the people one meets, accidents, world events like wars and natural catastrophes? Or is what we call free will perhaps only the way one faces or negotiates the journey imposed upon us? My grandfather's aura hovers again above me as I recall, from a beloved photo, the benevolent expression on his aged face. This irrational connection lends a very special mood to my mission.

～

One month before leaving for Afghanistan, the French Army sends me to spend two weeks of immersion in the British Army at York, in the north of England. I am supposed to familiarize myself with their military and medical protocols, which are different from our French ones. It's also an opportunity to meet Harry, the superior officer in the Royal Navy who will be my medical director at Camp Bastion. He is an anesthetist-resuscitator familiar with different kinds of war. In his fifties, of average height and robust, he looks at you with a frank expression and smiles easily. It's reassuring to know that this intelligent and sensitive man will guide my path in the theater of operations.

Every day, we rehearse and practice the motions and techniques of medical rescue systematically, for hours, during simulations of war situations. We all wear our uniforms as we will in combat. The only French person on board, I stand out because of my different uniform. Here I am, *l'exception française*—the French always like to think of themselves as exceptional.

The day begins at 6:00 a.m. and ends around 11:00 p.m. After a quick breakfast, we all meet up in the camp courtyard for the morning parade. Then comes an hour of marching at a military pace in the English countryside, which is often rainy. Back at the camp, we move on to the hard training in military medicine. The hospital is identical to the one at Camp Bastion. The equipment is the same, as well as its placement and disposition in the room, practically down to each syringe. Professional actors or veterans wounded in Iraq and Afghanistan play the roles of polytraumatized soldiers. A PA system broadcasts the sounds of helicopters and ambulance sirens, similar to what we will hear at the front. The atmosphere is strikingly authentic. The goal is for us to acquire the right reflexes so we can work automatically on the ground. It's also an opportunity for the doctors, surgeons, and paramedics to get to know each other, for they will work together at Camp Bastion.

On my end, it's another story. As a free agent, acquainted with no one, I spend a lot of energy integrating myself. I have to perform at a high level and assimilate as fast as possible the new concepts that the British call Damage Control Resuscitation, which I knew nothing about before my arrival. As the health service of the French Army hasn't trained me in the basic principles of military medicine, I have to figure things out for myself. As is often the case in France, you need some luck to get by. You have to roll with the punches and manage on your own!

My assignment is all the more difficult in that this mission was designed by certain politicians, and not everyone in the military supports it. There were some who would have preferred a career army doctor instead of incorporating and training a civilian. In both countries, they're watching me, and they let me know it. I can't fail.

I know I'm under constant observation. Superior officers are testing my resilience and my ability to cope under pressure by letting me understand that, because of my lack of experience as an army doctor, there's no chance of my getting deployed with the British Army. Fair enough. Conversely, from time to time, a curious character with a moustache, whose green beret suggests he could be an officer in the Royal Marines, comes to see and encourage me. "We need you, Doc. Hang in there, you've got to make this mission a success!" he says to me with a heavy Scottish accent, then disappears. My contact in the French Army repeats the same thing to me every time we speak on the phone. So I have someone on each side supporting me.

These trying days are periodically punctuated by sweet text messages from Clara. My training period is drawing to its conclusion when there's a bizarre incident. On this particular evening I'm relaxing in my room listening to Frank Sinatra singing "You Make Me Feel So Young" on my computer, when suddenly someone knocks at the door.

"Come in!"

"Hello. You're Elie, the French doctor?"

"Yes, I am!"

"My name's Peter. I'm a combat nurse in the British Army. There aren't any more free rooms because the camp is bursting with actors and extras for tomorrow's general rehearsal, before our departure. But I heard there was an empty bed in your room. Can I sleep here?"

"Of course you can, Peter!"

"I have to warn you about something, though. I've been suffering from post-traumatic stress since my deployment in Iraq in 2005. I was attacked by killer dogs trained by the enemy while I was saving one of our wounded men. My unit retaliated by firing and killing the animals. I was caught in the middle of the fight and almost died."

"And since then?"

"Since that trauma, every night between two and three in the morning I relive that ordeal as though in a trance. It'll probably wake you up. Don't worry if it happens."

"I see. It sounds like a kind of sleepwalking. And you've sought help for this?"

"I've tried everything—psychiatrists, psychologists, medication, psychoanalysis, behavioral therapies, hypnosis, EMDR, yoga, mindfulness—and nothing has worked. And my wife left me."

"Well, you can stay here. Anyway, you know I'm a doctor."

Later, around two in the morning, I'm woken up by Peter's night terrors. A full moon lights up the room. He's sitting on his bed, struggling in the shadows with who knows what demons. The scene is impressive, like a foretaste of what might be waiting for me at Camp Bastion. It's a night I won't sleep.

My room is on the ground floor of the barracks located at the end of the military camp and looking out on a garden. Early the next morning, like every day since my arrival, I'm getting ready for my morning exercise when, opening the curtains of the big bay window, I see before me an army of black crows at attention on the lawn, as though to recall the somber night just passed. For some reason, Laura's face comes back to mind.

Why did that woman appear in my life? What was she up to?

⁓

She had begun on a very personal note: "You're the professor who has inspired me the most. And you're Jewish, I think?"

Surprised by this direct and unexpected question, I answered her, "I inspired you because I'm a Jew and a professor? What a bizarre association!"

"No, mostly because of your compassion and gifts as a teacher. But I have a lot of affection for your people and attraction to it. When my father fell ill, my mother worked as a housekeeper for some Jewish bankers in London. They helped my family. I first went to Israel when I was seventeen; I've been back a number of times and have friends there."

I have to admit that, at the time, I was thrown off balance by this tall brunette with green eyes—by her self-assurance, spontaneity, and charm. I was about to agree to direct her university work when the Israeli services approached me. Then I had to leave the United Kingdom, and the relationship ended there—for a while. She reappeared later, for no clear reason. At the moment when I'd been entrusted with the mission to Afghanistan, she approached me again with her winning ways.

I received a kind of answer to my questions when I got back from York. Before I left for the Afghan war zone, I had to get clearance from the secret services of the French Army. Consequently, I was summoned by the DPSD, the security agency of the French Ministry of Defense, for an inquiry into my family, my friends and the people I'd met in recent years.

"That girl, Laura, landed in your life at the same time the Israelis targeted you?"

"Yes."

"We're going to get some intelligence on her because she may very well have worked for them."

"Strange, I'd never made the connection. But now that you mention it, she's been to Israel a number of times. So, you really think that—"

"Anything is possible! Those girls are trained for the job. They get to you through sex and emotion."

"For what purpose?"

"Intelligence. The Israelis wanted to recruit you and they weren't able to. Now you'll serve in the French Army and you'll be embedded in the British Army. That's enough."

"She would have been doing this for money?"

"You say she comes from a family of modest means, that her father got sick and that, to bring up her kids, her mother worked as an employee in the home of some Jewish bankers? In London, she was also one of your students at university?"

"That's right!"

"Then maybe she paid for her studies by doing some jobs for them. . . . We'll bring you up to date when you get back from your mission. From now until then, be prudent. For the moment, we advise you to be as neutral as you can."

There are still many gray zones regarding the nature of my meeting with Laura. Maybe when I return, the officers of the DPSD will tell me more. Should I really believe them? The world of intelligence is so complex and opaque. Truth comes packed in lies and vice-versa.

In the final analysis, Laura worked on me as a kind of electroshock, honing my defenses. I certainly needed that before leaving for the violence of war. Besides, I would never see her again.

～

The pilot's voice suddenly interrupts the stream of my reflections. "We are now flying over Central Asia. We'll arrive in Dushanbe in about an hour. You can adjust your watches. We are three hours and a half ahead of Paris time. It is currently 2:00 p.m. in Tajikistan."

9.
A SEASON IN AFGHANISTAN

The plane has just landed at the military airport of Dushanbe. I've barely stepped onto the gangway when a noncom calls out to me, "Captain Cohen? You're not going on to Kabul with everyone else. I've received orders from Paris. We're rerouting you through Kandahar."

"Are you sure about this?"

"I'm positive! Here is the order for your mission. You will take a military plane tonight at three o'clock in the morning in order to join a small French unit that's posted over there. They're the ones who will direct you on your mission to Camp Bastion."

It is almost 4:00 p.m., local time. It must be 12:30 in Paris. It's summer in Central Asia and very hot. We are standing on the airport tarmac with units of fighters and logisticians.

Dushanbe, in Tajikistan, is a base that functions as a gateway for a great number of French soldiers who will fight in Afghanistan. The US Army is present here, too. After a short briefing on the workings of the camp, we're given leave from barracks.

The base camp is situated at the airport in order to facilitate the movement of troops. It's very rudimentary. A small headquarters, a cafeteria for meals, a small internet room, common toilets and showers, tents for sleeping.

The internet is necessary for all these soldiers, who are deployed for six months far from home. In this kind of environment, stress and the sense of solitude are often hard to handle. It becomes crucial to speak to one's family, one's spouse, kids, girlfriend or boyfriend, and friends.

Our fathers and grandfathers didn't have all these amenities and comforts. They left for war, sometimes for years, without knowing when they'd come back. Many of them died. They could only communicate with letters. Hundreds of millions were written in 1914–1918. Contemporary conflicts are different. The new geopolitical situation, the use of satellites, computer science, and robotics have modified the old paradigms. The quality of logistics, equipment, clothing, hygiene, and food have improved at the same time. In this field, the Americans have always led the way.

Medicine has advanced and developed, acquiring better technical means and international protocols that have today been formulated by the Americans and British. However, France, with its long tradition of military medicine going back to Napoleon and before, still has its special areas of competence and excellence.

The other big difference is that our fathers and grandfathers were conscripts, therefore obliged to serve, with the threat of court martial if they deserted. In the present day, soldiers are professionals, committed and conscious of their choice to serve.

What hasn't changed is the environment with its consequences: death, and physical and psychological disability. The concept of posttraumatic stress disorder was developed in this context. French military psychiatry has a poetic term for these psychological traumas—"invisible wounds."

There's nothing new under the sun. During the Great War, there were already psychiatrists working in military hospitals to support the men wounded by the slaughter in the trenches and to keep them fighting, or to identify those who faked injury in order to avoid returning to the hell of war. In France, the psychological wounds of war, ignored for too long, were not officially recognized until 1992.

The new order of things also includes the incorporation of women into the army. There are many women in health services, administration, and logistics, and everywhere else as well. They rise to commanding positions. In some countries they can be found in combat. Historically, there have long been women fighters, infantry, and aviators. In the Red Army, for example, during World War II. The other side of the coin is that these Amazons can also be mothers. It's not easy to manage young children when you are a soldier deployed 3,500 miles from home. When you ask them why they decided to serve, they provide a moving answer: "In order to defend our children."

These situations are not easy to handle. Luckily Skype allows them to stay in touch and to see each other long distance. But there are limits to virtual contact. Fidelity as well. Military couples don't stay together easily.

~

At Dushanbe, the end of the day comes soon. It's always very hot. The airport is calm. I still haven't spoken to anyone. It's normal; I am the only one deployed "in isolation," as they say. The others are there with their units. They all know one other. And then I don't feel like communicating, I prefer to remain concentrated on my objective. In any case, the atmosphere isn't one for joking around. War isn't far away.

I've had time to locate my tent and put my kit down on an

empty bed. The air conditioning is rudimentary, but it seems to work. So much the better!

The internet café is full of soldiers, connected to the computers. I have to wait my turn for a little while before being able to look at my emails and send one to Clara and Paul, in order to reassure them I've arrived safely.

The dinner hour is approaching. I decide to take a shower in the meantime, while the toilets are empty and still clean. I haven't washed, shaved, or emptied my bowels in two days. It's best to do it now, all the more so because I begin at three o'clock in the morning. It's a life habit that I've always practiced, since my early years. To get ahead of the others in order to take advantage of space and hygiene. The sense of anticipation is fundamental in extreme situations. It's often a matter of survival. Once clean and lighter, I join everyone in the self-service cafeteria. The food is basic, but not bad. I sit across from two officers who want to engage me in conversation.

I remain laconic. I simply say that I'm a doctor, without going into the nature of my mission. The military rule being not to speak about it too much, they're not surprised, and the dialogue stops there.

Soon it's time to go to bed. Night falls quickly at this latitude.

Two thirty in the morning. Night has been short. Awakened by the alarm on my cell phone, I quickly get dressed by the light of my headlamp, which is indispensable in this environment, while trying not to wake the others up. Usually it provides light for me in the high mountains. We leave the shelters toward three o'clock in the morning with Eric, my friend and guide, in order to climb up the towering, silent peaks. I pick up my kit and head toward the military plane that should take me to Kandahar.

The previous night, I received a helmet, a bulletproof vest, and a first-aid emergency kit in case of a problem. Every soldier receives the same, consisting essentially of morphine to treat pain and a tourniquet to stop massive bleeding while waiting for rescue teams to arrive. Controlling hemorrhage is especially important if a limb is struck, as often happens in Afghan territory. All this gear, on top of my backpack, is beginning to be cumbersome. In its entirety, it weighs almost 90 lb.

Although it's night, it's still hot. I'll experience the sensation of dry and permanent heat during my entire stay in Afghanistan.

I make my way in the light of my headlamp. I quickly see the plane on the runway. Shadows appear around it. It's the unit of logisticians that I'm going to travel with.

"Captain, you're leaving in thirty minutes. Put on your bulletproof vest. You'll put on your helmet at takeoff. Do you have your earplugs?"

"Yes, in my bag, Sergeant."

"Get them out, you'll need them. There's a lot of noise in military planes and helicopters. In war you have to take care of your eyes, ears, and . . . feet. A soldier who can't walk well is no longer a real soldier!"

"So I've been told."

"I see you have good shoes, perfect for the desert. They're Blackwalks, aren't they?"

"Yes! They were recommended to me before I left," I say. In fact, I heard they would be more suited for the desert than French shoes, especially if I have to wear them full-time for two months. I also have special desert eyeglasses, American as well. "Listen, I don't have any weapons besides my survival knife. Is that normal in a theater of operations?"

"Normally physicians in the military health services don't carry them, except in the commandos. Most of the time, they're working in the military hospital in Kabul where they're relatively protected. Moreover, given their lack of training, they're rarely a good shot and would be more dangerous with a pistol than without. . . ."

"I agree, Sergeant, but I'm going to be deployed in isolation in the theater of operations, traveling alone for a great part of my mission, and maybe even evacuating the wounded in hostile territory!"

"I grant you that. Did the army teach you how to shoot?"

"So to speak. My only military training took place during a fifteen-day course with the Marine Commandos, during which they tested my basic physical condition, my adaptive capacities, and my medical knowledge. The rest, I did by myself, because of personal inclination."

"What do you mean?"

"I had a hunch that the army intended to send me some place on a foreign operation. So I worked on getting in shape and on shooting as a sport. Luckily, when this mission came through, people in the Special Forces took me in hand and intensified my training."

"How did you come into contact with them, Captain?"

"I've given up trying to figure that one out. Let's say they were connected to the shooting club where I was training. They arrived at the right moment. Maybe the army was behind it, but there's no way of knowing. I think I was lucky, that's all!"

"Fortunately you understood that you could only rely on yourself. I have no worries about you. They gave you a certificate of your ability to shoot in war zones, I suppose?"

"Yes!"

"Once in Kandahar, ask for a handgun. It will be useful for you to have one at Camp Bastion."

"Regarding my temporary rank of major, when do I put it on?" I'd been given an extra stripe for the mission.

"I see, they gave you a fake promotion. You'll put it on before you join the British. In their eyes, you'll be more credible in the guise of a major. For the moment, have a good flight and good luck with your mission, Doc! You're expected at the Kandahar airport."

"Thank you, Sergeant!"

The military airplane resembles those I've already seen in the movies. It's used for the transportation of troops. You enter it from the back and the interior is vast. Backpacks and the soldiers' other equipment are piled up in the center. On the sides, along the whole length of the cabin walls, there are folding benches where we sit in the half-light. Around forty soldiers, including a few women. In the front, the cockpit with the pilot and copilot. In the back of the flying machine, two sentinels are posted standing before the portholes. One on the left, and one on the right of the aircraft, behind their machine guns, ready to retaliate in case of enemy attack. I'll learn at Camp Bastion that the insurgents are in possession of missiles and rockets, and that flying in the Afghan sky is dangerous. Flights are often made at night. Security necessitates it. Planes take off almost vertically, taking altitude quickly in order to get out of range of attack, as the enemy has missiles that can only reach planes and helicopters when they are within the limited range of taking off or landing.

We put on our helmets and bulletproof vests before departure. In observing the way the others are dressed, I see, as I suspected, that they didn't give me a uniform appropriate for summer. I'm surely going to be very hot in the Helmand desert.

The sergeant was right, the motor makes a lot of noise. No one is talking to anybody. In any case, it would be hard to hear each other. After a day and a half of traveling, having barely slept since our departure from Paris, we are all very tired. The pressure gradually increases. Soon, we will be in the theater of operations.

10.
KANDAHAR

Kandahar and its military airport. It's five in the morning. The trip lasted an hour and a half, without any complications. It's already daylight and hot out. The air is dusty.

After having recovered our bags, we wait to go through the security check. In Afghanistan, the protocol is the same for all flights: on departure as on arrival, compulsory passage through a systematic and careful search. A logical procedure, for in this war without a front line, suicide attacks are the main danger.

Outside, a young, aspiring French army doctor stands in front of a 4 x 4, waiting for me. His name is Dominique.

"Hello, Captain. Welcome to Kandahar!"

"Hello, you can call me Elie."

"We only learned of your arrival yesterday, without really understanding what you've come here to do."

"I have to say it's really unbelievable, to find no one expecting me after a journey of almost four thousand miles from home, without any plans for getting back!"

"So sorry, but I am not in on headquarters' secrets. I do find it strange, in fact. Come, I'll take you over to the French quarter."

Like all American bases, the one at Kandahar is immense. While we drive along, Dominique tells me about himself, his daily life since he arrived here a month ago.

"Here we're just a small unit. Most of our troops are in Kabul and in the valley of Kapisa Province. The team of maintenance technicians for the air army, which you just traveled with, has come to relieve the previous one. They'll take care of the Mirages and Rafales. You'll also see soldiers from the Special Forces and intelligence. Our little community clinic takes care of the health of all these fine people. I have two regular nurses and one auxiliary nurse assisting me. We mainly do general medicine and take care of minor injuries."

"And major emergencies?"

"The American hospital at the base is in charge of those. They have state-of-the-art services, including in neurosurgery."

"This is your first experience on a foreign operation, Dominique?"

"Yes, I had a stroke of luck. I finished my studies only a year ago. When they suggested I leave for this posting, I accepted immediately, though I'd just gotten married. It's harder for my wife than for me."

"You're here until when?"

"Until December."

"I understand your wife. You talk about getting lucky, but do you really feel that way?"

"The goal of every soldier is to serve his country. That's what I'm doing here. I'm a little envious of you, Elie."

"Why?"

"Because you're going to zones on the front lines where combat will be intense. It'll be grueling, but truly rich in unique experiences. For a civilian doctor, it's not a common situation!"

I'm not sure that every soldier's goal is to serve his country.

There are different reasons people join the military, and not all are patriotic. Some are there because it's a job, others for the adrenalin or the adventure, and so on. Dominique is young and inexperienced, fascinated by the myth of war. I understand his intellectual interest in the special cases war presents to medicine, but I think it's important to question the reasons for war and to remain lucid and critical. War is sometimes a necessary evil, but one should also ask who—which powers, businesses, individuals—are going to profit from this?

As I listen to Dominique, I gaze at the desert landscape and the vast spaces where the camp is located. It's hot and dry. The sky is an intense blue.

"What's our altitude here?"

"Around three thousand feet. You see those mountains towering above us?"

"They seem rather far away."

"Not as far as you might think! The insurgents often use them to launch rocket attacks from their peaks. When the alert sounds, we take refuge in the bunkers. If there isn't enough time, we get down on the floor on our stomachs. I'll explain the procedure to you. . . ."

Along the way, we pass buildings belonging to the NATO countries involved in this conflict.

"So this is an international base?" I asked.

"Yes, Elie. It was originally American, but all the countries of the international coalition are now present. I think we're now actually managed by the Canadians. I'd need to verify that."

"How many men and women are actually serving in Afghanistan?" We are, in 2011, in the tenth year of the war.

"In the larger contingents, there must be around a hundred thousand Americans, ten thousand British, and five thousand French. Then there are representatives of the other fifty NATO nations."

We are walking along the enclosure that protects the camp from the outside, beyond which I suddenly spot the tip of a minaret that reminds me I'm in a Muslim country.

"What's behind the wall?" I say, gesturing toward the concrete wall with barbed wire. I'm disoriented since my arrival at the airport. "How far are we from Kandahar?"

"About ten miles. It's an important urban center. The second in the country with around five hundred thousand inhabitants. Did you know it was founded by Alexander the Great in the fourth century BC?"

"I read that when I was getting ready for my trip. And also that many cultures have passed through here in different historical periods. The Greeks, Indians, Persians, Mongols, Arabs, etcetera."

"In fact, the Silk Road connected the West to China with a narrow band of territory that was forty-seven miles long, located in the northeast of the country."

As he talks, my eyes wander back to the minaret, and I feel doubly out of place, not only as a civilian thrust into military life, but also as a Jew stranded in the middle of a Sunni Muslim republic. And it's a complicated country with thirty-four provinces and a number of ethnic groups. Helmand Province is located near Pakistan and Iran. The major ethnic group here is Pashtun, which is also the dominant ethnic group of the whole country and the one that the current president, Hamid Karzai, belongs to, as has often been the case with Afghan leaders.

We finally reach the French headquarters. I have the feeling, probably from fatigue, that we've been driving for a long time. The spot is quiet. Its surface area isn't large. It consists of a few buildings, with the administration and recreation center in the middle. I quickly take a tour of it with Dominique before meeting the director.

"Hello, Doc," he greets me. "I'm Colonel P___, responsible for this unit of the air army. Welcome to the base! I have to admit that twenty-four hours ago I wasn't aware that you were coming. Apparently HQ at Kabul wasn't either. It seems that Paris informed them at the last minute. I don't understand anything about this business . . . Anyway, you're here, so we'll deal with your situation. So, you're going to Camp Bastion?"

"Yes, Colonel. I'm going to be working there as an emergency doctor with the British in order to bring back a report for our health service."

"I heard you're not a career military man. So what are you doing here?"

"Everybody's been asking me the same question, and I always give the same answer! I suppose they chose me because of my dual nationality, French and British, my experience in the health systems of both countries, as well as my training as an emergency doctor in the French service. As for why else, I have no idea. Maybe also they just couldn't find anyone else for the job."

Years later I'll learn that, as a consultant—in other words, a kind of mercenary—I cost less than a professional soldier because the French Army would have less of a pension to pay me in the case of my death. And if I'd died, the media wouldn't have been obliged to cover it.

"Destiny, then—if you believe in it."

"We'll see. . . ."

"Fortunately you're physically fit, Doc, because you'll need to be. Dominique gave you a quick tour of the camp. Now he'll show you the medical office that's located elsewhere, near the maintenance area for our planes. We get our meals in a cafeteria shared by all the armies of the coalition. For the moment, we need to arrange your departure for Camp Bastion and your return from the mission. When are the British expecting you?"

"As soon as possible, Colonel!"

"You have their contact information?"

"I only have the name of my medical director there. I met him before my departure, during my training in England. Do you have his phone number at Camp Bastion?"

"No, you'll have to get it from the British infirmary at the base."

"The army was supposed to have organized all this!"

"Typical of the French! They get you in a mess, and then you have to figure things out for yourself!"

"They already did that during my deployment. The French noncom in charge of my dossier didn't speak English. I had to contact the British Army myself to set up the logistics for my trip. I even had to pay for my Eurostar ticket, my first nights in London, and the train to reach my training camp in the north of England. And right before I left, they realized I didn't have my security clearance. I finally got clearance at the last minute; otherwise nothing would have been possible."

"It all sounds familiar, Doc. Complete chaos, and then the struggle to get out of it. The French Army will reimburse you!"

"I hope so! When I consider how disorganized they are, I start questioning what I'm doing here. I don't really feel like going any further, not that I have a choice at this point."

"It's possible they were trying to protect you by waiting till the last minute to announce your arrival. This is a very dangerous country, you know. You're traveling by yourself, so it's better that troublemakers know nothing about it."

"For reasons of security . . . You really believe what you're saying? Even if your hypothesis is true, it still remains the case that this mission is my responsibility, and they're leaving me on my own to sink or swim. I'm even going to have to call Camp Bastion myself to rejoin the British Army. To top it all off, I'm not even armed. That's travelling light in a war zone, don't you think? I'd kind of like to stay alive."

"I understand you, Doc. But now that you're here, you have to see the thing through. We'll help you. Go see the logistics officer of our camp to contact the medical director at Camp Bastion and organize the departure for your trip there. I'd advise you to arrange your return in advance, because you'll pass through here again before rejoining the French forces in Kabul and going on to France."

"I should arrange my return now?"

"Yes! Reserve a place in the military plane that will take you back to Paris. If you miss that one, you might have to spend another month in Afghanistan waiting for the next. You'll also get a handgun that you'll return to us when you come back from your mission. I hope I've been clear. See you later."

As I'm leaving the colonel, an alarm is sounded for a Chicom. We take refuge in one of the camp bunkers, not far from there. Chicoms are the Chinese-made rockets Dominique has told me about. They can fall anywhere. Those who haven't had the time to reach a shelter have gotten down flat on their stomachs. Every man for himself!

While waiting for the end of the alert in the concrete tunnel we're using as a bunker, I reflect, perplexed, on the situation. How could the military authorities have deployed me with such apparent amateurism? This mission seems to spring more from a political agenda than a military one. That's perhaps why everything has been organized at the last minute. Suddenly, I recall what the noncom in charge of my dossier said to me, "I don't understand who decided to deploy you in Afghanistan. Not long ago you were blacklisted because of your contacts with the Israelis. Because of that, you never should have gotten a security clearance. And in your case, it would be impossible for you to leave for this war zone without it. It leads me to believe that they must really have needed you to change their minds a hundred and eighty degrees!"

I also remember my meeting with a French colonel from head-quarters, right before my departure. "You have carte blanche!" he said. "Once you're with the British, try to work at all the emergency stations. You'll be writing up a report for us on their care of wounded soldiers. It seems their protocols are innovative."

"Will I also be going into combat zones to pick up the wounded?"

"Yes, of course! In helicopters, with the MERT," he says, referring to the Medical Emergency Response Teams.

"You're asking me to take a lot of risks without my having received sufficient training. It's all pretty incredible, if you ask me. I find it hard to believe that you haven't been able to find an army doctor for the job."

"I have to admit, there was a lack of clarity around your deployment. But this mission was put together so fast that we didn't have the time to organize it correctly. And then, it's a pilot project with everything else still to be figured out. Only a bicultural guy like you could succeed here. Sorry your name was the first to get picked out of the basket!"

"That's easy for you to say! Another thing, Colonel, the medical director of Camp Bastion, whom I met during my training with the British Army, was astonished by my rank of captain. He was expecting to see a lieutenant-colonel. He suggested I be made a major to make my mission more believable in the eyes of his colleagues, once I get there."

"It's too late for us to officially name you major, but we will 'zinc' you for the needs of this mission."

"'Zinc' me?"

"Yes, it's a classic procedure for a deployed soldier. For the purposes of a special mission, we give him a rank above the one he holds. When he returns, he returns to his old rank."

"I see, and I'll be paid as a major?"

"No, as a captain, your real rank."

"Obviously. How stupid of me—"

"In fact, you won't see me again, I'm about to be transferred to a new post. You'll have to hand in your report to my successor."

What nice speeches from this member of the top brass, who seems to care about his own image more than he does soldiers in the field. He'll surely gain a star if I'm successful. Perhaps that's why he's so interested in my mission. This time, I definitely understand that I'm the only one I can count on. From now on in, I'll have to take charge of everything myself.

~

A little later in the day, I go to the British infirmary at the Kandahar base because I'm trying to reach my medical director at Camp Bastion. A nurse, to whom I've explained the reason for my mission, kindly helps me place the call:

"Hello, Harry?"

"Elie! Where are you? We're waiting for you. We were beginning to think you'd gotten lost somewhere in Afghanistan!"

"I'm in Kandahar. What do I need to do to join you? The French haven't arranged a connection for me!"

"Bloody French! Listen to me, every day there are British military planes linking Kandahar to Camp Bastion. Go contact our HQ in Kandahar, choose a flight with them, and keep me posted. I'll send someone to greet you on your arrival."

~

In the late afternoon, back at the French camp, I'm approached by an officer from the DPSD. In his thirties, small and dry, dressed in jeans and a T-shirt, the officer speaks to me with the detached manner typical of intelligence professionals.

"I was expecting you. Paris has just briefed me on the purpose of your mission at Camp Bastion. I'll be your contact in Afghan territory. The job of the DPSD is to protect you. Here's my cell phone number. If you have the slightest concern or any doubts about any of the people around you, call me."

"I find it reassuring that someone is finally aware of my presence here!"

"Are you supposed to do medevacs from combat zones?"

"It's a possibility, according to what was suggested in Paris."

"Good. You'll also need a weapon. A pistol should do it. Go see the armorer; he'll give you one, and ammunition, too. You'll turn it back in when you come back through here from Camp Bastion. I'll see you at that time to get a first report on your mission. I've nothing more to say. Good luck, and be careful!"

～

Later, in the cafeteria, seated with a few French soldiers, I get into a conversation with a man of the cloth. He's a tall, strong-looking guy, with a direct, smiling manner; he wears a chaplain's collar under his military uniform.

"I'm a Protestant chaplain for the armies. You're leaving on a mission with the British, Doc?"

"Yes, my plane leaves tomorrow at four in the morning. And you, Reverend, what are you doing here?"

"I'm here to care for suffering souls!"

"There must be a lot of them in Afghanistan!"

"Yes, Doc. We've just lost several soldiers."

"I heard about it. It's important to have a spiritual presence and a man of God in an environment like this one."

"You're direct; we like that where I come from, in the territory of Belfort!" he says, referring to an area in the east of France, not far from the Jura Mountains.

"I know, the people in that part of the country are tough, Reverend. Some of my partner's family are from there."

"You have to be resilient to go to war. Extreme situations can trigger religious feelings in an individual. In a theater of operations, stress, disability, and death are permanent realities. In this context, one becomes acutely aware of human fragility. We men of faith are here to answer the questions that come up."

"Those questions often have no answers. . . ."

"In that case, our role is still to try to soothe the torment experienced, even if one feels powerless when confronted by certain situations."

"Your words are humble and honest, Reverend. I don't know if we'll meet again, but I'm glad we had the opportunity to talk."

"I'll be in Kabul when you return from your mission. We'll speak again of such things. In the meantime, may God protect you."

~

Back in my room I think about my parents. They're elderly, so I have to stay in touch with them regularly and continue to protect them by hiding from them the truth about what I'm doing. My cell connects to the local network, and although it's forbidden to make outside calls, I decide to dial them, after concealing my location on the phone. In France, it's early evening.

"Hello Papa! Is everything okay in Paris?"

"Yes! Where are you, Elie?"

"I just arrived at my friends' house in Switzerland. We're leaving for Austria in a couple of days. I told you, we're going to do some hiking for a good part of the summer. It'll probably be hard for you to reach me in the mountains. Don't worry about me. I'll call you from time to time to keep you posted."

"When are you coming back?"

"At the end of the summer. This year I'm taking a long break. After three years without a vacation, I really need it because, on top of everything else, when I get back I go straight to London."

"You're still working in London?"

"Yes."

"So we won't see you soon?"

"It'll be the end of September before you know it. And I'll be calling you once or twice a week!"

Hanging up, I experience a wave of guilt. But I have no choice; these lies are the only way I can spare my aged parents. My father, whose health is fragile, wouldn't be able to handle my departure for this Afghan war. He knew World War II, his father had been in the one before that, and one of his brothers fought in Algeria. I don't want to add myself to the list.

Too much, it's too much. . . .

11.
CAMP BASTION

Two thirty in the morning the following night. Dominique accompanies me from the barracks of the French sector to the airfield.

"You need time to get through security, and then boarding takes an hour. Your flight is scheduled for 4:00 a.m. Put your gear in the back and get in the car. Here, I've got some water and fruit for you if you want some. You have to stay hydrated. Drink often and in little sips. Even at this hour of the night, it's hot."

"Yes, the nights aren't always cool in the desert, as I'd expected. In any case, thanks. You were very efficient in helping me resolve the problems I had because of the sloppy way Paris HQ prepared my deployment."

"Everything is, a priori, taken care of. There weren't any more summer uniforms in your size, but we've got you a Beretta nine millimeter with two magazines and ammunition."

"Okay, that's not much, and it isn't a recent model, but at least it's a good one. In any case, as the armorer said, joking, if they come after you with a machine gun, clear out and run!"

We soon reach the airport. A lot of soldiers are waiting at the entrance. There must surely be a delay for security reasons. Boarding will take two hours.

The RAF plane carrying us is a Hercules. I'm with British and Americans. Around thirty men. As was the case during the trip that took me from Dushanbe to Kandahar, we're sitting on red folding benches that run against the outside walls for two-thirds of the length of the cabin.

At the rear, our backpacks and military material are heaped up and restrained by safety ropes. This time, on top of the two sentry-men standing in the classic manner on either side of the plane, a third one stands before the rear hold, his hands on his machine gun battery, ready to fire at the slightest danger. The mood is tense. In Afghanistan, a country of mountains, the air network is used mostly for the transport of troops and wounded. In spite of the risks, it's less dangerous and quicker to move around this way than to travel by road.

Respecting the protocol, we all put on our helmets and bullet-proof vests, and insert our earplugs. I'm the only French person in the group. Unlike me, the other soldiers are wearing lightweight, camouflage-print uniforms suitable for the hot, dry climate of the Helmand desert in summer. The British ones are khaki beige. The Americans wear gray-green. Mine is khaki green, elegant but intended for the mountains of the northeast of the country, rather than the desert of the south. Bad fashion choice, General!

Soon it's six in the morning. We have reached our destination. It's day and already hot. The sky is eternally blue. Here the mood strikes me as different. To my great relief, I don't have to go through any security check, the main part of which has already been done in Kandahar. So much the better.

Camp Bastion is located in the southwest of the country, in Helmand Province, a desert plateau that stretches out at an altitude of around 3,000 feet toward Pakistan and Iran. Although it's very dry, Helmand is crossed by a river of the same name. Coming from high, mountainous peaks, it surges through the middle of the desert and irrigates many poppy fields. For the British troops, it's the end of the road. Beyond it is the front without a front, in other words the FOBs—forward operating bases—the Green Zone and its drug traffickers.

At the exit of the military airport, an athletic young blond woman waits for me, standing in front of her Jeep in full sun. She nods to me. I'm easy to spot because of my French uniform. Smiling, she addresses me with the gentle detachment characteristic of certain Englishwomen. "Hello, I'm Captain B__, but you can call me Leslie. Are you Major Cohen?"

Suddenly I'm a major and no longer a captain. I wonder whether she has been informed of my "zincing."

"Yes, that's me. But call me Elie, please."

"Welcome to Camp Bastion, Elie. I'm one of your colleagues, an emergency physician in the Royal Navy. They've put me in charge of taking you to the hospital and helping you out for the day. Come, throw your stuff on the back seat, and get in the front with me. Have you had a good trip from Paris?"

"The flights went well enough, Leslie, but there were hitches in the planning. Normal, I suppose, in war zones?"

"That depends. The British units come directly from Oxford. It's precisely in such situations that one needs to minimize the risks by carefully preparing deployment down to the last detail. From what Harry told me, that doesn't seem to have happened in your case?"

"That's right. The trip ended up being broken into stages. From Paris to Dushanbe, from Dushanbe to Kandahar, and from

Kandahar to Camp Bastion. Most of the time, solo. It would have been better if I'd flown directly from Oxford, under the protection of the British Army. But forget about it. The important thing is that I'm finally here. I hope my mission goes well. The camp seems really huge."

"It's our largest base for foreign operations since World War II. We built it in 2006. More than twenty-eight thousand people live here, including ten thousand Brits at Camp Bastion itself, and eighteen thousand Americans at Camp Leatherneck, right next to us. But there are also Danes, Estonians, Georgians, Pashtun interpreters, as well as maintenance teams, which are mostly Filipino. Not counting the five thousand Afghan soldiers posted at Camp Shorabak, not far from us."

"And the hospital?"

"It's very busy. Half of the personnel are British, the other half American. We work well together. Our protocols are similar. You'll see some difficult cases here, but you'll also have a unique experience."

I discover Camp Bastion along the road we're taking. Leslie explains the place to me as she drives. I learn that there are four zones, Camp Bastion zero, one, two, and three, which have gradually developed since 2006. Its structure is simple and efficient. Traced on the model of American cities, its roads are laid out at right angles, and between them are rows of air-conditioned beige canvas tents. The buildings with "hard" construction are reserved for HQ, superior officers, and VIPs, for the military training zones, sites of worship, cafeterias, surplus stores, a few cafés and pubs, and the hospital.

Life at the camp is in full swing starting very early in the morning because of the heat. Along the way, we cross paths with US Marines, British Royal Marines, maintenance workers, and armored military vehicles returning from mission. Further on, along annex roads, Chinook and Merlin helicopters are landing and taking off.

"So here we are. This is Role 3 hospital. Come, Harry is expecting you. Then we'll go to your room so you can drop off your things."

A hospital is designated Role 3 when it is located at a main camp and is capable of the most advanced care. Role 1 refers to first aid on the field, and Role 2 to a light structure close to the field where you can provide basic surgery.

We catch Harry walking toward us.

"Good to see you, Elie!" he says. "You've finally joined us. I was wondering if you'd ever get here."

"Me too, Harry!"

Leslie leaves to go back to her duties in the emergency department, and Harry takes over the tour.

"I see your commanding officers added a major's stripe since your training at York. A good thing, it'll make your mission more viable."

"It's temporary, and there's no salary increase coming with it! I'll go back to being a captain on my return."

"I'm familiar with this kind of procedure. Not really fair play on their part because you deserve the rank of major, Elie!"

"I cost them less this way. . . ."

"An officer from your HQ is going to reach the base in the late morning to meet you. After all your adventures, I imagine he wants to make sure you've arrived safe and sound at Camp Bastion."

"Better late than never. . . ."

"In the meantime, your true mission is about to begin. I'll take you on a quick tour of the hospital and introduce you to the teams, especially the emergency doctors you'll be working with. Then we'll talk about the organization and your schedule. Then you can go rest. You must be tired after your long trip."

"You bet! I need a little break before I start working."

"You'll start treating patients only after having observed us operate for a couple of days. You've already seen many of our methods when you were at York. There shouldn't be any problems."

"You know, while we're on the subject, I've had the impression of being out on my own. But now the success of my mission depends on all of us."

"We're aware of this, Elie. We know it's your first experience of war and that the French system is different from ours. You can count on us. You'll work at all the different emergency positions, most of the time joining teams that take charge of polytraumatized soldiers using Damage Control Resuscitation."

"And the medevacs of the wounded?"

"You'll do a few, by plane or helicopter. You should know, however, that we may not be sending you into certain extremely sensitive zones."

"My superiors gave me carte blanche to go everywhere. . . ." I feel frustrated. If I'm going to war, I should be full in for the whole adventure. And that was what the French Army was expecting.

"We know your commitment, don't worry. You'll be doing more than you imagined and, above all, we'll make sure you get to go home safe and sound. Come, we'll put your weapon in the safe."

"Why can't I keep it with me?"

"That's the protocol for health workers at the hospital. The only armed doctors are those who go pick up the wounded from combat zones. You'll get it back if you do evacuations from combat zones."

"It's strange, Harry; I feel like I already know this place."

"That's a good sign! It proves that your training in the UK was productive, since the hospital at York where you prepared for your mission is a duplicate of this one."

"An example of famous English pragmatism!"

~

From 2006 to 2008, the hospital was located under a huge air-conditioned tent, ready to function in the event of a massive influx of wounded. The one I'm in now with Harry was built in 2008 by the British Army. The structure of this prefabricated building supports speed of execution, which is crucial in the context of extreme medicine. It extends at length, one single block without any upper floors, an immense open space where you can move rapidly from one service to another. Thus, the emergency department, radiology, lab, surgical block, intensive care, and blood bank are all connected in real time. Like all elements of the camp, the hospital is air-conditioned because the temperature outside can reach 122° F.

Two hundred and fifty people work there night and day with all the technical and modern facilities of a London or Paris hospital at their disposal. The medical staff, logistics, and administration are drawn half from the Royal Navy, half from the US Navy. These are complemented by teams from the RAF and the US Air Force. I'll also meet several Danish doctors because their Special Forces have been fighting in the area.

The emergency workers, intensivist–anesthetists, orthopedic, visceral and vascular surgeons, nurses, paramedics, and combat medics are all dedicated nonstop to the care of the soldiers. In this extremely hot environment, hygiene is crucial and remarkably well attended to, for the prevention of iatrogenic infections is a top priority. The maintenance technicians and cleaning crews are working continually. The smooth operation of the air conditioning and machines is essential. Heat and dust constantly create problems.

"Here, we're cursed by exploding mines, Elie. Soldiers come in without legs or arms, or even worse. You'll also see blasts, wounds made by bullets and grenades, military vehicle accidents, and little traumas as well as common medical issues."

"What about the local population?"

"We care for the Afghan army and police, as well as some members of the population, such as children mutilated by the mines, which they mistake for toys. Their hospital stays don't last more than three weeks."

"What happens to them afterwards?"

"After that, they're transferred to Afghan hospitals. Unfortunately those places are real death dens because of the poor training practitioners receive here, the lack of means, negligence, and iatrogenic infections."

"They need to get better, then, during their stay here . . ."

"I forgot, we also take care of prisoners. As is required by the Geneva Conventions. And then they are important, for reasons you can understand," he says. I guess he's referring to their possible contribution to intelligence gathering.

"Your logistics are impressive."

"It's based on an essential principle: speed of execution. I suppose you've heard of the 'Platinum Hour' and the 'Golden Hour'?"

"Yes, Platinum for the first ten minutes of a medical rescue and Golden for the hours right after. They're crucial for survival and for recovery. The concept of rapid rescue came out of World War I."

"Like triage, which is, as you know, a French expression. We're in the desert, near the front lines. A helicopter evacuation takes an average of fifteen minutes from the combat zone to the emergency services."

"Where do the wounded come in?"

"The landing strip for the helicopters that bring them back is located just two hundred meters from here. We hear them land while we're getting ready to receive patients. The ambulances take five minutes and park right in the entrance that connects directly to the emergency ward, where we immediately take charge of them."

I already know that medevacs and frontline hospitals date from the Korean War. The M*A*S*H*, or Mobile Army Surgical Hospitals, were medical–surgical antennae. These structures, linked to the use of helicopters, increased the speed of intervention and therapeutic success, as well as the use of plastic pouches for blood transfusions. Although it is difficult to compare what isn't comparable, during the First World War, 45 percent of the wounded died; during the Second the number dropped to 35 percent. The numbers dropped again, to 24 percent, during the Korean and Vietnam wars.

"Today in Afghanistan," my guide continues, "we only have a 10 percent mortality rate. The 'Bastion Way' is unique."

"The 'Bastion Way,' Harry?"

"Camp Bastion is the busiest place in the world for the poly-traumatized. Last month we did more blood transfusions than they do in a year in Scotland!"

"Incredible! Where does the blood come from?"

"75 percent of fresh frozen plasma, red blood cells and platelets come from the United Kingdom. The remaining 25 percent comes from the US."

"And whole blood?"

"We draw it from our soldiers in Afghanistan," he says. "They've all been tested before their deployment; we know their blood type, and we know they're healthy. The lab techs play an important role in this, given the massive quantities of blood required for Damage Control."

"That makes sense."

"That's what has enabled us to experiment and develop cutting-edge rescue protocols that we've called the 'Bastion Way.' I know that the goal of your mission is to become familiar with our methods and to write up a report for the French Army."

"Yes, Damage Control Resuscitation and Damage Control Surgery. Everyone was talking about it during my training in England."

"Exactly," Harry says. "Everything begins in the combat zone with the stabilization of the wounded, the rapid intervention of the MERT, and the blood transfusion that is started in the helicopters."

At Camp Bastion, the MERT are the military emergency rescuers of the RAF. Two teams, each composed of one anesthetist or emergency doctor, one nurse, and two paramedics, are continually on duty. Men and women, these war zone saviors evacuate in record time those soldiers wounded by the insurgents.

Unlike the French SAMU, which employs doctors in the pre-hospital civilian emergency services, the British use paramedics for that function. These health care professionals have training in emergency protocols and procedures. Capable of infusing and intubating, they waste no time on the ground and get the patients very rapidly back to the resuscitation areas or trauma centers. This is the famous "scoop and run" developed by the Anglo-Saxons and Israelis.

"I see the emergency department has ten resuscitation rooms."

"Yes, if necessary we could take charge of six critically poly-traumatized at the same time."

Next door, opening onto the emergency department, I can see the operating block with its four operating tables used nonstop for Damage Control Surgery. Behind the bloc is the intensive care section with thirteen beds for recovery. Adjacent to the emergency entrance is radiology with its two latest-model CT scanners. Then a little further on, one after the other, the laboratory and blood bank.

"Where are the hospital beds?"

"We have thirty of them in two internal medicine departments located toward the middle of the building, behind the recovery area."

Going down the long corridor, we pass the hygiene and infectious disease departments, then we finally reach the general medicine service that the British call Primary Care.

"You've been a practicing physician in the United Kingdom, so you know that Primary Care centers are at the heart of our system. They include general medicine, dentistry, mental health care, physical therapy, and treatment for STDs."

"Although sexual relations are officially prohibited in the armies. . . ."

"Theoretically, yes. But in reality, things happen, and we have a specialized nurse who takes care of that area. Physical therapy, rehabilitation, and manipulative therapy are located inside the tent that previously served as a hospital until 2006."

In the camp, hundreds of soldiers consult Primary Care doctors every week, essentially for classic general and preventative medicine. The practitioners, including dentists and physical therapists, also move into the zones closest to the front. Besides caring for the seriously injured, the British Army is very attentive to the comfort of its young fighters, as the morale of the troops and their physical hygiene are two necessary conditions for the proper conduct of a war like this one. As I listen to Harry, I think again about 1914, about the massacres during that war and the soldiers who fought then. A soldier's life then was not precious to his commanders the way it is today.

Located in a building facing the hospital are the administration, the offices of the Royal Air Force and the US Air Force, as well as the MERT department. To top everything off, there's a little chapel, built on the outside, which is used for celebrating Anglican and Roman Catholic mass.

"The RAF and US Force," Harry says, "organize helicopter

medevacs, transport into the military hospitals of Afghanistan and their repatriation to Europe. The serious polytraumatized cases don't stay in Camp Bastion for more than forty-eight hours. British soldiers are rapidly evacuated in medevac planes back to the Queen Elizabeth Hospital in Birmingham in the UK, and American soldiers are provisionally transferred to Landstuhl in Germany before being transported to the military hospital in Washington, DC."

"How long does the transfer back to England take?" I ask.

"Around eleven hours. An intensive care team goes along with the wounded. For security reasons, the C17s fly at night," he says, referring to planes especially equipped for the purpose.

"All this has a price tag."

"War is expensive! Moreover, we have to have the permission of adjacent countries to fly over their territory."

"I can imagine the kind of deal—"

"And now it's time for you to take a break, Elie. You'll eat with Leslie, then she'll take you to your room. You'll start work tomorrow. From now until then, you're off duty."

A few minutes later, I find Leslie, and we walk toward the cafeteria. In the desert, at this time of day, the sun is very hot and the light intense. It's absolutely necessary to wear a desert hat that protects both the head and the back of the neck, as well as UV protection glasses and sunscreen. The difference in temperature between the air-conditioned interior of the hospital and the outdoors is dramatic. During my time at Camp Bastion, I'll walk the eight hundred meters between the hospital and the cafeteria again and again, and each time in a bath of heat and dust. The two dominant colors—the blue of the sky and the dark beige of the sand and tents—will be impressed on my memory for good.

"Elie, has Harry given you the schedule for your work shifts and professional meetings?"

"Yes, briefly. He simply told me that when I'm not doing night shifts, I'll be working every day in the emergency ward from seven in the morning until eight at night."

"Every morning at eight, there's a meeting of the entire staff with Harry. Representatives from all the departments—doctors and surgeons, nurses and administrators—attend it. It's to discuss the patients and logistics."

"Just like in a traditional hospital."

"Then at eight p.m., the doctors and surgeons meet again for an informal meeting to review problems that came up during the day."

"Okay."

"Every week, phone conferences are set up between the health personnel at Camp Bastion and those at Queen Elizabeth Hospital in Birmingham and the American Landstuhl hospital in Germany or the military hospital in Washington, DC. They're used to follow up on the wounded who have been transferred."

"Understood."

"Other weekly meetings are organized for professional updates, as well as presentations of statistical studies regarding the organization and efficacy of the care given by our teams. Don't worry, you'll get a day off from time to time."

"The only thing left for me now is to start work. . . ."

We reach the cafeteria, which is in a large shed. There is a place to wash your hands at the entrance; hygiene is obligatory. We get on line to use one of the two rows of sinks. Inside, at mealtime, the place is always filled with a crowd of British soldiers, a few Americans, some Danes, and the Filipino workers contracted to take care of the camp's maintenance. I'm the only Frenchman. Surprisingly, the food supplied by the army, a mix of Indian and English cuisine, isn't bad. A well-fed soldier is an important thing. In order to avoid dehydration, rations of water in small plastic bottles are placed at our disposal and stored in huge, easily accessible refrigerators. Water is a precious resource, to be used as needed, but not wasted.

We join some of the emergency physicians I'll be working with during my mission: another British one named Sharon, and three Americans, Jimmy, Robert, and Sam.

Robert turns to me with a humorous expression.

"You've come from the land of Lafayette!" he says. "You've delivered us from the English, and we saved you from the Germans. *Lafayette, nous voilà!*"

"That's one way of looking at it! We helped you at first, and vice versa, and now it's your turn to lead the dance."

"How long will you be with us?" he asks.

"Six to eight weeks, depending on how things go and my ability to integrate myself into your team."

"The British," Sharon says, "will do everything they can to support you, Elie. You're already one of us because you've worked in the UK. And you even have British citizenship. Your mission will surely be successful."

"I hope so, Sharon, but that isn't enough. I have to show my worth on the ground. . . ."

12.
IN THE HEAT OF THE HELMAND DESERT

Somewhere in the Helmand Desert. It's nine thirty in the morning. The helicopter has just left the British base of Camp Bastion for a medical evacuation.

It has to be done very fast. It's an absolute emergency. An A-level priority. The confrontation, in the Green Zone, was violent. The patrol fell into an ambush. One of the soldiers stumbled on a mine that the enemy detonated from a distance. He was seriously wounded, and the prognosis for his survival looks poor.

Including the time taken to check the medical equipment and arms, it took the team less than eight minutes to get into a flying machine and take off. It's a Chinook. A CH-47. It belongs to the mythic line conceived by Boeing and used by the US Army in the Vietnam War. The Royal Air Force uses the Chinook to transport troops and to evacuate the wounded. Its size is impressive. When its khaki cabin moves through the skies with its two propellers whirring, one in the front and the other at the rear, it looks like a giant insect that has stepped out of the dinosaur era. As though war were sending us back into prehistory. . . .

On the inside, in the shadows, the pilot and his copilot, the MERT, and the infantry soldiers at their protective posts behind their machine gun batteries are ready to intervene if attacked. Every movement in the Afghan sky invites danger. The rebels have ground-to-air missiles they use when the helicopters are in range—that is to say, when they're taking off or landing. Standard equipment for everyone includes helmets, bulletproof vests, anti-UV sunglasses, ear plugs to mute the noise of the helicopter, HK assault weapons, and 9 mm Sig 226 pistols.

From the moment I arrived at Camp Bastion, I felt immediately connected to the MERT. In this team I found the spirit of the SAMU that I knew so well. These saviors have been trained for combat. Here, the so-called rebels zap the Geneva Conventions. It's a victory for them when they hit a doctor or a nurse, a way of weakening the troops' morale. A soldier is reassured by the knowledge that he'll be taken care of in the event he's badly wounded. It supports his efficiency. The enemy's tactics are vicious, but logical. War gives "permission to kill." Doctors and nurses are there to minimize the collateral effects of this legalized violence, but they must know how to defend themselves as well as how to save lives.

~

The flight has lasted fifteen minutes. The helicopter is about to set down in the combat zone, in the desert, in the middle of nowhere. Major Rob signals his men to stay ready. A doctor anesthesiologist, he's the officer in charge of the MERT. Tall, blonde with blue eyes, he has a manner that is both straightforward and flexible, in the way of Englishmen of his breeding. He has natural authority.

The din of the motor and propellers makes communication

difficult, but everyone knows his job. The rear door is completely open. The heat and dust are intense. Four infantry soldiers exit quickly to secure the zone. Mike, one of the paramedics, goes next. The other members of the team remain on board, because the risk of being taken down by a sniper is too great.

At the same time, the first-aid workers of the unit in question approach with the wounded soldier on a folding stretcher and help get him on board. The maneuver is not supposed to take more than ninety seconds. That's the recommended maximum amount of time in order to minimize the risk of being hit by the enemy.

At first glance, everyone understands that this polytrauma-tized soldier has minimal chances of survival. The man is in a coma. When it exploded, the mine cut off his two lower legs above the knees. The testicles have certainly been hit as well. His right forearm has been half torn off. Tissues have been burnt, some to a cinder. The pelvis and abdomen have also been damaged.

On the ground, the combat medic and other soldiers have already removed his helmet to free his upper breathing passages and to put in place a cervical collar so that any eventual vertebral fractures will not be aggravated. They have placed tourniquets on each thigh, close to the wounds, which they stuffed with compressive hemostatic dressings intended to slow or stop bleeding; then they treated him for pain with a morphine injection. The medic uses a random piece of paper to improvise a record sheet with notes on the type of wounds and initial clinical data. They are succinct.

The young fighter is still breathing, but with difficulty. His condition is unstable. The carotid pulse is present, but the radial pulse cannot be felt. As a consequence of the blast from the explosion, he must still be bleeding abundantly in the thorax and abdomen, because he's very pale. The remaining portions of his extremities are marbled and cold. His oxygen saturation level and blood

pressure are very low. He's in hypothermia. His heart is beginning to show signs of suffering on the monitor. His Glasgow
Coma Score—a system used to indicate level of consciousness—is
at three, the lowest possible, and his right pupil is a-reactive and
dilated, indicating serious cerebral damage.

There isn't a moment to lose. Even if the case seems like a lost
cause, one must try everything and stick to the protocol for hemorrhagic shock. Everyone around the patient is involved. Care
measures are begun as the racket made by the helicopter taking
off once again makes it hard to hear, so verbal communication is
supplemented by sign language. The lack of comfort and light are
unimportant. The scene is harsh.

Major Rob directs the operations. He prepares the intuba-
tion kit while Mike and Jim, the two paramedics, prepare the
sites for the intraosseous infusion, one in each shoulder and the
third in the sternum. Phil, the nurse, will inject the resuscitation drugs at those sites. Ketamine and Celocurine for intuba-
tion; ketamine again for pain; Fentanyl for sedation; Augmentin
to prevent infection; tranexamic acid to slow down bleeding;
red blood cells and plasma warmed to body temperature. The
blood transfusion is massive. That is the key treatment, its
goal being to fight against a triad of killers: hypothermia, aci-
dosis, and coagulopathy. This is the famous Damage Control
Resuscitation, dear to the British. The patient is finally intubated, ventilated, and transfused.

The return trip takes a quarter of an hour, during which the
condition of the patient deteriorates in spite of the management of
respiratory passages and the massive transfusion. He dies as soon
as he reaches the hospital. His name was Greg. He was twenty-four
years old.

Everyone at Camp Bastion is dismayed. Rob addresses us:
"We'll have to announce this soldier's death to his family in

England before the media get involved. Communication networks will be cut temporarily."

~

I say to Rob that death was the best possible outcome for this soldier. Wouldn't life have been unbearable for him without his legs, with his testicles damaged and only one functioning arm? Rob agrees, but then his training as an army doctor takes over. "Your point of view is defensible, but ethically, we are obligated to try to save everyone. And then one must avoid deaths on the ground. Western public opinions requires—"

"Dirty devices, those IED's," Mike interrupts, referring to improvised explosive devices. This red-haired Scotsman is squarely built and likeable. He has already served in Iraq. Visibly moved by the situation, he continues his explanation. "These damn mines are very destructive and the cause of most of the big combat injuries. They're homemade or collected in the zones abandoned by the Russians after the war they lost against the *mujahideen* in the 1980s. The goal of the insurgents wasn't to kill, but to seriously mutilate troops in order to deal a blow to the morale of soldiers and Western public opinion. This is also a war of nerves and propaganda. Their technology is constantly improving thanks to allied powers."

"Which ones?"

"Pakistan and China," Phil answers from behind his technician's eyeglasses. A wry smile masks his anguish. "These devices are detonated from a distance. The enemy uses mobile phones to set them off, and they explode when the soldiers are coming through."

"One mine can also conceal another," adds the sturdy Jim. His cockney accent is typical of what might be heard in East London, and his blue-green gaze goes straight to its target. "The

British troops know this well because of where they've landed. The Helmand is our theater of operations. One of the hardest in Afghanistan. Our soldiers are young. They're under orders to apply the counter-insurrection strategy the Americans have dictated. Make war against the insurgents and peace with the population. That's the new doctrine installed in Afghanistan by NATO's chief of operations, General Petraeus."

I nod, having learned during my training that the inspiration for this theory came from David Galula, a French officer, now deceased, who specialized in guerilla warfare. Threatened by the Nazis during World War II because he was Jewish, he joined the Resistance, then the US Army under the orders of General Patton. In 1949, stationed in China as an intelligence agent, he observed the insurrectionary tactics employed by Mao, which would later be used against the French Army in Indochina and Algeria.

"Who are these insurgents, Rob? Are they all Afghans?"

"It's a melting pot, Elie. Most of them are Taliban descendants of the Pashtuns, a dominant ethnic group in Afghanistan. Taliban means 'student of the book.' These Sunni fundamentalists come out of the Pakistani Koranic schools, real brainwashing machines. In 1893 the British drew the Durand line and divided their territory, Pashtunistan, into two parts. One sector is the area here in Afghanistan, south of where we are now, and the other is in the tribal zones in the north of Pakistan, which provides support as part of a deep strategy intended to provide security in the event of a conflict with India. The Pashtuns are at the same time clamoring for unification, which doesn't improve matters any."

"And the others?"

"They belong to Al Qaeda and those fighting in the movement for international Muslim integration, rallying to intensify jihad against the crusaders that we're supposed to be. They come from

Chechnya, the Middle East, the Horn of Africa, the Maghreb, France, the UK, and elsewhere."

"I understand, especially since the NATO coalition includes almost fifty nations."

"Yes, it's a world war of a third type, a war in which religion plays a predominant role. Not only with Muslims but with extremists of all kind. They fan the fire."

"But why is the fighting localized here?"

"It's an American war, Elie. Central Asia presents big geopolitical stakes. Afghanistan has always been a corridor between Europe and Asia via the Silk Road. For Russia, it provides access to the warm seas. Iran and the Persian Gulf aren't far away. There are huge gas and oil reserves in some of the surrounding countries and in the Caspian Sea. Right now people are talking about rare metals in the Afghan earth. Not to mention opium. . . ."

"Opium?"

"Around ninety percent of the world's heroin comes from Afghanistan. The Green Zone, where we went to get that poor soldier, contains one poppy field after another, extending to the horizon toward Pakistan and Iran, through which most of the trafficking passes toward Europe, Russia, and the USA. The mafias and the arms traffickers are also involved in this big game."

"The British have also fought here, Rob?"

"Yes, three times between the nineteenth and twentieth centuries. These confrontations pitched the British Empire against Russia, which fought each other to acquire sole control of the region—the famous Great Game. Today, the Americans are taking a turn. Whoever controls Central Asia controls the world. This requires a subtlety that Texans don't always cultivate."

"Which maybe explains the quagmire we're in today?"

"Partly. During the Cold War, the USA supported the Afghan

mujahideen against the Russians, and then they supported the fundamentalist Taliban, joined by Bin Laden. For thirty years Afghanistan has been a reservoir for modern jihad."

"The Americans are fighting them right now!"

"That's right. Commander Massoud, whom the French liked a lot, paid the price with his life when he was assassinated by terrorists two days before nine-eleven. Since the end of the Cold War, the world has returned to the geopolitics we inherited from World War I."

"The Sykes-Picot Agreement?"

"Yes, the division of the Ottoman Empire drawn up by French and British diplomats. Many of our contemporary conflicts have come out these agreements, in which one of the stakes was oil."

~

While Rob talks, I remember the discussion we had with Shimon in Jerusalem. Once more, I wonder who's going to benefit from all this. How can Westerners imagine they might make peace with these populations whose countries they've invaded once again? History seems to repeat itself in another manner, as though obeying a law of recurrence. Two different civilizations look at each other without understanding. But there's no time to question what we're doing here, for the team, on duty until tomorrow morning, has to leave again for another rescue operation. Two Afghan children have been hit. They must be evacuated rapidly. In spite of their failures and the harshness of situations encountered, the MERT love their job and are always happy to save lives whenever they can.

Because someone has to do this job. War has never been clean, though the Yankees would like us to believe otherwise. Today like yesterday, the doctor at the front is there to relieve the suffering of victims. In the past hundred years, the shape of conflicts has changed. At the beginning of the twentieth century, approximately 80 percent of the wounded and lost were soldiers. Today, 80 percent of victims are civilians.

This is the era of wars that are permanent and without any front lines.

13.
ARMY MEDICINE

Five o'clock the next morning. My alarm rings. Opening my eyes, I see the light of dawn through the opaque glass of the skylight that serves as my only window. My roommate still seems to be asleep. His name is Bill, and he's one of two internists in the British health service deployed at Camp Bastion. Our room resembles a ship's cabin. It's small, long, painted white, and air-conditioned. A bunk bed, two desks, and two chairs are the only furniture. For security reasons, openings to the outside are limited, and most of the time we use neon lighting to brighten the room. The atmosphere is spartan. Our pale gray, prefabricated barracks are surrounded by anti-mortar cement walls. Located not far from the hospital, our quarters shelter the British and American teams of doctors and surgeons who are lodged two or three to a room. Men and women are separated, their bathrooms, too. The Filipino workers in charge of maintenance are scrupulous in their attendance to hygiene.

I get up without making too much noise and go straight to the bathrooms. Ever since my arrival, two months ago, I've stuck to the same morning routine, being one of the first to wake up in order to take advantage of toilets and showers while they're still clean. Back in my room, I find Bill awake and getting ready to go for his morning jog. You have to go running very early at Camp Bastion because the heat gets intense fast. Bill is a big blonde guy, around thirty years old, always smiling and a straight talker. A career army doctor, he's on his second tour of duty in Afghanistan. His mission is to guide me and facilitate my integration into the team by helping me with daily problems, and he's doing it well.

"Hi, Elie," he says. "Last night, when I came back from my shift at the hospital, you were sleeping so soundly I didn't want to wake you."

"Yeah, it was an intense day. I was so exhausted I just fell into bed. I'm running to get breakfast. I'll see you at the hospital."

The cafeteria is right next to our barracks. Breakfast is served from 6:00 to 8:00 a.m., lunch from noon to 2:00 p.m., and dinner from 6:00 to 8:00 p.m. After a rapid English breakfast, I join the emergency service. It communicates directly with the ambulance area, at the entrance to the hospital.

Twenty-four hours a day, seven days a week, three members of the medical staff, with different specialties, rotate every eight hours. Harry is already ready to go with his emergency personnel.

"Hello Elie, did you sleep well?" he asks.

"Like a baby, I was totally out."

"Good! We're expecting a serious injury in fifteen minutes. He stumbled on an IED. According to MERT," he adds, "he has lost at least a leg and a hand."

∼

We hear a helicopter landing on the strip nearby. Suddenly everyone looks serious. We all know that in a few minutes we'll have to

act, and fast. In the moment, I am one with these teams of ultra-
competent doctors and nurses who are caring and strong at the
same time. Harry has made sure that my integration has gone
smoothly and the training I got in York is serving me well. This is
no place for sentimentality, which can only get in the way of efficiency. Our only goal is to save whatever is salvageable. One often
has to go into a dissociative state in order to tolerate the horrific
sight of these mutilated men, some of whom have flesh shredded
by land mines.

But there's no time for reflection, for MERT is already there,
transporting the wounded man on a green khaki stretcher with an
iron frame. In their British army uniforms, harnessed like fighters
with bulletproof vests, helmets, and assault weapons strapped on
their shoulders, they're covered with desert dust, their faces wet
with perspiration from the heat and the rush of adrenalin.

The protocol begins. It's impressive, always the same, as strictly
ruled as sheet music, and it unrolls like a true psychodrama in an
almost religious silence.

The MERT doctor, assisted by his nurse and two medics, begins
by giving us a detailed clinical description of the patient's condition and the measures taken during his evacuation. He has already
transmitted some of these facts during the helicopter transport
via secure satellite telephone. A nurse has noted them down on
a board hung on the wall, near the resuscitation room right near
us. With this protocol, used for maximum efficiency and speed of
execution, everyone is already aware of the details of the case.

This soldier is British, twenty-six years old. He was patrolling
on foot when the mine exploded. He's covered with blood. His
right leg has been ripped off just under the knee. His right hand
has also been injured. After being anesthetized, he was intubated
and ventilated, and he received a blood transfusion. The smell
of human flesh hit by explosives is intensified by the heat of the

climate. I'm having a hard time getting used to it, and I confess I still smell it now as I write these lines.

On the ground, the protocol for the management of hemorrhagic states of shock has been applied, as usual. The combat nurse has placed a tourniquet on his lower limb and, at the same time, stuffed the wounds with hemostatic dressings. With these tourniquets, developed by the Israelis, you simply have to turn a kind of handle attached to the straps to tighten and compress the tissues in order to stop the bleeding. During the helicopter transport, the MERT started resuscitation and succeeded in stabilizing the wounded soldier.

Trapped in this war, in this extreme situation, I find myself facing all the big questions about the human condition. Life and death, suffering, handicap, hate and violence, love, too.

And God in all this?

The Devil, for sure!

The exploitation of ignorance and religion. The collision of different civilizations. Geopolitics, economic interests, the business of war, the mafias and trafficking of many kinds, including opium and heroin, all in some crazy melting pot. Why did this boy, barely out of adolescence, have to come to Afghanistan and lose his leg, far from his country, in this bloody war? He could be my son. He'll be handicapped *ad vitam aeternum*. This human sacrifice seems insane and is part of the sordid game we've embarked upon.

In the meantime, one must act to save him. The resuscitation continues. Two teams are on site. The first consists of the actors using the defibrillator, the wounded soldier on his stretcher, and the medical personnel, myself included. The observers are in the other group—an evaluating team composed of emergency doctors, anesthesiologists-resuscitators, surgeons, male and female nurses, and members of the administration. They stand apart in the little hallway that connects the emergency area to the operating theater, behind a yellow line drawn on the ground which they mustn't cross. From behind this symbolic border, they analyze our management of the wounded. Their notes will serve to improve protocols. It's a reflective process.

On the other side, the drama unfolds in silence. The mood is meditative, almost religious, because death is never far away. Concentration is at a maximum. A little schizoid, I continue to split myself into two in order to tolerate this hyper-realistic situation and to put my humanity at the service of this wounded soldier. The best way is to concentrate on one's task and gestures. Elie, the army doctor, has become a technician devoid of the emotions that a normal being would experience faced with this scene. There's a sense in which my state is subordinated to the team that's focused on saving this life.

About twenty doctors and nurses are gathered around the victim on his stretcher. About half are British and half American. There are as many women as men. All are wearing their summertime military outfits: canvas pants, T-shirts, and Rangers. On top of that, they wear a lead vest covered with a light green plastic apron designed to protect them from X-rays and blood. They have their latex gloves on and protective eyeglasses. I'm wearing the same gear, but in the colors of the French Army.

In a war zone, the concept of asepsis exists, of course, but it's slightly different from what you might see in the emergency services and surgical wards of European and American hospitals. In this environment and these very special circumstances, things pass that wouldn't be allowed in a civilian context. Only efficiency and results count. And it works.

We're in the second stage of the Damage Control Resuscitation protocol, the first having been started by the MERT on the ground. It's the British who developed this protocol specific to Camp Bastion. Everything is meticulously coded. Large quantities of blood have already been ordered. The priority is to minimize the collateral effects of hemorrhagic shock.

The soldier is transferred from the stretcher to the resuscitation room while being checked for the presence of other wounds, and the treatment begins. The measures are rapid and precise, executed without panic. A real ballet, coordinated by the emergency doctor at the foot of the stretcher; he's the Primary Survey Doctor and the true orchestra conductor directing the proceedings. He oversees the operations, but doesn't participate in them directly. In the event of a large influx of wounded troops, an anesthesiologist-resuscitator or a surgeon can take on this role. Everyone knows what he or she has to do. One gesture per doctor or nurse. The sequencing of tasks reminds me of Taylorism—scientific management—applied to medicine: we function as a medical assembly line.

The anesthesiologist-resuscitator and his anesthesia assistant, who is not a doctor, stand right next to the polytraumatized patient. Their usual job is to introduce a tube into the respiratory passage and a catheter into the central venous system. In the present case, the patient has already been intubated in the helicopter. His ventilation is functioning well. So they insert the central catheter in order to replace the intraosseous infusion.

To their right there always stands an emergency doctor, the Secondary Survey Doctor. While looking for secondary wounds that haven't yet been listed, he tracks the clinical state of the victim and his vital signs. Today, that's my job. I don't find any secondary injuries.

Also present are nurses, paramedics, combat medics, and medical auxiliaries. One of the nurses helps me put a pelvic binder on him in case there is abdominal bleeding. Others take charge of infusing, injecting resuscitation drugs, and transfusing fractions of human blood using machines, called Level One, that propel under pressure pouches of red blood cells, fresh frozen plasma, and platelets that have been warmed to 107° F. This enables the rapid refilling of the victim, who has already lost a lot of blood and needs to be treated for hypothermia.

The radiologist and his technical assistant are positioned behind me. They are ready to do the thoracic-abdominal-pelvic X-rays and a FAST (Focused Assessment Sonography Trauma) scan, which will be interpreted on the spot. They don't find any bleeding in the abdomen or thorax. The so-called runner is in charge of blood and the laboratory tests. He's the liaison with the doctor lab technician. The surgeons (orthopedic, vascular, visceral, and plastic) are already present in order to evaluate the state of the wounds and to plan the surgery.

Next to the Primary Survey Doctor, a scribe verifies and documents that all the procedures have been followed properly. Each member of the team announces when his or her task is done. This medical-legal information will be used in statistical studies in the field of military medicine.

From behind the dividing line, Harry and the members of the administration survey the resuscitation room. They are prepared to organize the return of the soldier to his country of origin or, in the eventuality of his death, to inform his family. In the latter case, the communication between the camp and the civilian world will be cut off until his next of kin is notified, so that the morbid press won't get wind of the news beforehand.

Once the clinical state of this young soldier has been stabilized, he's rapidly transferred to radiology for an entire body CT scan, in order to identify any associated internal lesions, including brain damage. We always do this with polytraumatized patients. The entire attending team, still focused and silent, accompanies him in a cortège toward the radiology department. This procession has a sacred feeling.

He will then go to the operating theater for hemostasis and cleaning of the wounds, which is called Damage Control Surgery. Since the arrival of the MERT, the treatment of the patient has taken twenty-five minutes. All together, the process of his transport from combat zone to the surgical table has taken less than an hour. He will survive, after the amputation of his right leg and his hand on the same side, and will be transferred forty-eight hours later to England, destination Queen Elizabeth Hospital of Birmingham.

~

Afterwards, Harry gives me a look of solidarity tinged with helplessness.

"I have to admit I still find it hard to process all these horrors," he says. "But one must cope."

"What will become of this soldier without his right leg and his right hand?"

"He'll be a different man from now on. His life will never be the same. Once back in his country, he'll undergo more sophisticated surgery in order to get him ready for prostheses. Then he'll get reeducation."

I ask him where the center for reeducation for military personnel is located.

"Headley Court is in the outskirts of London," he answers. "Wounded, handicapped patients get great care there. Our rehabilitation programs are very proactive. The quality of the prostheses are constantly improving. As you know, these days you can do competitive sports minus one, or even two legs."

"And is there a limit to follow-up care? Do they receive benefits?"

"For three years, and then everything stops. They continue to receive a pension and to get care from the NHS," he says, "but they're removed from the army. At least they receive a

lump sum to help set up a home environment for the handicapped. That's the least that can be done! Strangely enough,
their ability to pull through isn't necessarily linked to the
severity of their handicap. As always, some will manage better
than others, but the majority will remain deeply affected. A
loving family can help a lot."

"And if they don't have support?"

"It can become an ordeal that takes them straight to hell."

"Why save everyone at all costs?"

"It's an ethical question."

"Aren't there also political considerations?"

"What do you mean, Elie?"

"Public opinion and the European media are globally against
the war, so it's better to avoid fatalities. As for the wounded, well,
we can talk about them later. . . ."

I feel Harry stiffen. I understand that, as a soldier for the Queen,
he must maintain a certain discretion, so I don't insist.

He answers as best he can: "Afghan children wounded by
mines have an even crueler destiny, Elie! Often the mines explode
in their hands when they're playing with them. If they survive,
these mutilated kids have a tragic future, because their society
rejects the handicapped. They've become useless to their families
and society, so they end up beggars."

∾

Once the rescue operation has been completed, the drama is over,
and everyone goes back to join his respective service until the next
polytraumatized soldier arrives, which happens before the day is
done. For many soldiers are transported to Camp Bastion on a
daily basis. A continuous flow of seriously wounded troops, with
legs, arms, and sometimes testicles ripped off. There are simple,
double, even triple amputations. On average, three to four a day,

not counting other emergencies. It's a full-time job. I don't know if I'll ever be able to erase from memory the images of these inanimate bodies, covered with blood and deformed by explosions. Real chunks of meat, bad-smelling, with burns ready to rot, for the heat of the climate doesn't help. I'll have to learn how to deal with sensations and flashbacks that I guess I'll have for the rest of my life. That's the lot befalling those who have known traumatizing situations.

I often imagine my colleagues, the British physicians in World War I, who had to take care of thousands of victims at once. The first day of the Battle of the Somme, there were around sixty thousand wounded, of which almost twenty thousand died. How did they manage? It was impossible to save everyone. Many were dead in the fields. The practice of triage was born at that time.

In Afghanistan, the risk is constant and affects everyone. Outside the camps—at the checkpoints, in the villages, and on the roads—danger lurks in the form of mines and ambushes. On the inside, we are exposed to suicide attacks and mortar fire. Helicopters taking off and landing can be the targets of missiles and rockets.

The goal of the rebels isn't only to kill, but also to strike at the morale of the troops and their families, as well as public opinion in Europe and the United States. When one has few means, as is their case, morale and propaganda are elements of strategy.

In patrolling the Green Zone, the young British soldiers follow American strategy. Caught in this trap, they get hit by improvised explosive devices, the infamous IEDs.

Ironically, these are made with the fertilizers that the United Nations supplies to peasants in order to support the development of the country's agriculture. The way to hell is paved with good intentions. In order to make these mines more harmful, the insurgents combine the misappropriated substances with bicycle pedals and goat dung, bits and pieces of which turn up in the soldiers' mangled limbs. In a paradox of guerilla warfare, the enemy, who's fighting with bare feet and a Kalashnikov, uses modern technology in the form of the mobile phone to set off the mines. These devices do a lot of damage, both on a physical and a psychological level.

In this hostile context, it's important to keep a watchful eye on the soldiers' mental equilibrium in order to locate psychological dysfunctions as early as possible, for the sooner these are taken care of, the better the outcome will be. Everyone at Camp Bastion has received a little booklet that explains the first signs of disturbance. If someone notices a behavioral change in one of his fellow soldiers, he must report it immediately. A psychiatric nurse manages the first symptoms. Trained in behavioral techniques, he employs EMDR. Eye Movement Desensitization and Reprocessing seems to yield good results, as long as it's used soon after the traumatizing incident. This behavioral treatment, a kind of hypnosis developed at the end of the eighties by the American psychologist, Francine Shapiro, is implemented by the British Army in its management of post-traumatic stress. These techniques may be helpful in the short term, but the effects of war trauma can manifest themselves for years. Over the long haul, verbalization and analysis seem indispensable.

Freud and the psychoanalysts understood this with World War I. French military psychiatry followed the same path in recently developing the concept of invisible wounds.

Those working in health care don't escape the stress. Ready to attend to seriously wounded soldiers 24/7, they are, by the very nature of the situation, constantly confronting war and its collateral effects.

Physicians, nurses and stretcher-bearers on the front line must above all do their duty while always being aware that their own lives are in danger. This requires not only professional competencies, but also courage, commitment, and self-control. Members of the medical staff on the front line are trained like warriors because they provide a privileged target for the enemy, who knows that wounding or killing one of them will deal a blow to the morale of the troops he is fighting against.

∽

Back in the emergency department, I see Leslie, the British emergency doctor, again.

"You're back just in time, Elie," she said. "There's a fair amount of small traumatology waiting for us. A military vehicle got turned over on one of the rotten roads in the area. We have to take care of a dislocated shoulder, a tibia fracture, another fracture in the forearm, and two minor cranial injuries. There's also this American soldier who put a bullet in his own thigh while handling his weapon. . . We'll divide up the work."

As a rule there's a great sense of solidarity among the different medical teams. There's no feeling of hierarchy; the only thing that counts is one's function. The protocols have been well honed.

The unit runs like a huge labyrinthine machine. Seven emergency physicians (myself included), four visceral surgeons, four vascular, a trauma surgeon, and a plastic surgeon; to which one must add sixteen anesthesiologists, two resuscitators, two internists, two doctor lab technicians, supported by four lab workers, three general physicians, two dentists, three physical therapists. Then there are the nurses, operating assistants, paramedics, combat medics, auxiliary mental health workers, the nurse in charge of hygiene, the interpreters, the Catholic priest, the Anglican pastor, the athletic coaches, two teams of MERT composed of four members each, the maintenance, cleaning, and medical staffs, the administration, the

RAF, the US Air Force and their sanitary airplanes for evacuation, and the rest of the logistics team. In this extreme context, all available energy is oriented toward the patients. As health professionals, all are inured to the trials of human suffering. Humor is also a valuable tool. It's a good remedy against the blues.

In addition to the major wounds of war, the unit takes care of small traumatology and accidents of all kinds. Just as in any European emergency unit, we sew up gashes, apply plaster casts and splints, and treat dehydration, sprains, sciatica, kidney stones, and all kinds of infections.

The presence of a plastic surgeon is specific to the health service of the British Army. It's a sound idea. His role is to advise the other surgeons on the way of treating damaged tissues. His knowledge of plastic surgery enables him to foresee how certain scars will evolve, with most of the wounds in this dirty war being amputations that will have to be equipped with prostheses down the line. His experience and long-term vision are essential. Because they know that plastic surgery and preparation for prostheses will follow, rescue workers on the ground place the tourniquets as close as possible to the wounds in order to respect the healthy tissues around it.

Camp Bastion is, in a certain sense, a frontline laboratory, a place of experimentation for the future. Americans have invested millions of dollars in neurosciences, nanotechnologies, and mechatronics. Artificial limbs linked to the brain by sophisticated, miniaturized digital systems, true intelligence prostheses, will enable paraplegics and quadriplegics to walk again with exoskeletons. And in a more distant future, one can imagine an ability to cultivate, from stem cells, tissues that would enable the reconstruction of muscles, bones, even organs, through the practice of autografting.

In the midst of the afflictions they create, wars have always led to advances in medicine and surgery. That's the positive side of these dramas. The First World War saw experiments in blood transfusion, in surgery to repair damaged faces, and in neurosurgery. Then, resuscitation and antibiotics came into being during the Second World War.

The longer I stay at Camp Bastion, the more I understand the role that the French Army has asked me to play here. I'm immersed in a true laboratory of wartime medicine. The experiments conducted here, to which I'm a privileged witness, will lead to new techniques and innovations that will most likely be applied in civilian hospitals in years to come. Perhaps the report I'll make to the army will serve that purpose. In other words, I have come into this hell in the service of humanity. Seen in this light, my mission takes on another meaning and, in the moment, seems more useful to me.

As the Buddhists say, "It's in the mud that the lotus grows."

14.
LIFE AT THE CAMP

Camp Bastion is in surface area as big as the city of Bordeaux, that is to say almost half the size of Paris. In 2011, it's the center of British military operations in Afghanistan. It's a true desert fortress, almost impenetrable, surrounded by eighteen miles of wire fencing and thirty-six watchtowers, in each one of which about five men are permanently keeping a watch over the insurgents' movements, with the help of a hundred surveillance cameras. This British base, the biggest one since World War II, cost almost a billion euros to build. Every day, six hundred airplanes land and take off from its airport, which is as busy as London's Gatwick. Three thousand vehicles, many with heavy equipment, circulate on its roads.

Ten thousand British soldiers and four thousand civilians live in over twelve hundred air-conditioned tents. The superior officers and VIP have the right to individual rooms, which are basic but comfortable and located in "hard" buildings. They all have toilets and television. Certainly very different from the precarious conditions of the worldwide conflicts of the twentieth century.

All in all, the fighters are well housed, they shower every day, they can do their laundry in the washing machines, and they have access to recreational areas. Sexual relations, alcohol, and illegal drugs are officially prohibited, but in real life things can happen.... Sports, which can compensate for sexual scarcity by providing an outlet, include jogging, cardio training, weight lifting, boxing, and martial arts. Men and woman train together under big air-conditioned tents, to the rhythmic sound of booming music.

Money circulates in the virtual form of cardboard tokens fabricated by the British Army and for use in Camp Bastion only. Soldiers can use them in the supermarket to get toiletries, T-shirts, chocolate bars, and sodas; at the corner pizzeria to buy a pizza; at Starbucks, or at the pub where they can have nonalcoholic beer with their buddies.

The internet and telephone networks are secure. Thanks to prepaid, inexpensive cards, soldiers can communicate with their families and friends in the UK in reserved spaces equipped with computers and phones. Skype works full throttle. BFBS, the local radio station, broadcasts daily programs of entertainment for the troops. *Good morning from Camp Bastion in Afghanistan*—it's good for morale!

Certain buildings are dedicated to the soldiers' training. They have even reconstituted an Afghan village in one corner of the camp. Inhabitants from the area play themselves in order for the fighters to familiarize themselves with their way of life. The camp organizes simulations of combat against fake Taliban to sharpen guerilla reflexes before actual deployment in the Green Zone.

The base is built over an enormous aquifer that springs from the mountain ranges in northern Afghanistan, the highest of which, the Hindu Kush, reaches 25,000 feet. In the summer, it's one of the hottest places on the planet. Temperature can go as high as 122° F. An enormous amount of water is consumed; it's used for the soldiers' personal consumption, as well as cooking, washing, and maintenance. Since 2006, millions of quarts have been drawn. There is on location a real plant, functioning 24/7, for the treatment and bottling of water issued from this aquifer. Workers from Sri Lanka and Nepal work there. Samples of water are sent every week to the United Kingdom for analysis of its purity and quality.

This industrial water treatment complex belongs to KBR, a subsidiary of Halliburton, the American company that is said to have close ties to Dick Cheney, later vice president of the United States. You can't stop business.

The same goes for food. For security reasons, such as the possibility of poisoning by locals, it is imported from the United Kingdom and the United States by plane or boat, via the Mediterranean and the Persian Gulf as far as Karachi in Pakistan, and then by road. Between 2006 and 2014, three immense cafeterias have served millions of meals. Every week, 27 tons of fruit salad, 7.5 tons of French fries, 105 tons of meat and fish, and 66,500 eggs are eaten. Here too, private companies participate in and benefit from these huge logistics designed to nourish over thirty thousand souls.

I'm two-thirds of the way into my stay and haven't had a moment to kick back. Since the beginning of my mission, I've been working hard to integrate myself into a system I didn't know, while being weighed down by the heavy, permanent atmosphere of war.

Searching for spirituality in the middle of this violent universe, I had a moment of wanting to speak to a man of God. As there's no synagogue in the camp, I found myself at Catholic mass on Sunday morning with a band of fervent Filipinos who were singing "Our Father" accompanied by guitar. May the Good Lord forgive me for attending, but you can't find a good rabbi when you need one! And after all, Jesus was also a Jew!

Given the exhausting work that takes up most of my agenda,

there's little time for recuperation, reading, or exercise. My day begins at five in the morning with a bit of gymnastics and yoga. When I'm not on duty, I fall asleep around midnight. Outside of the hospital, I try to gather notes taken on Damage Control and the protocols of the British health service in order to write up the report I'm supposed to hand in to the French Army. My idea is to get going on it while I'm on site and my memories are fresh.

I'm communicating regularly with Clara and Paul via internet. I avoid telling them about the horrors I'm seeing here in order not to worry them. Similarly, when I use the camp's secure line to call my parents, I continue to lie to them, letting them believe I'm in the Tyrolean Mountains.

The magic of music softens the most inhuman places. A few days ago, I went to a concert given in the camp by professional musicians serving as paramedics in the British Army's health service. The quality of their performance was remarkable. As I found myself outside, in the night and the desert heat of this country at war, with all these soldiers listening to an orchestra playing Gershwin, Bach, Purcell, and the Beatles, I felt like I was in a mirage. A little emotion can't hurt in this hell in the middle of Central Asia.

I'm getting along well with Bob, my roommate. He is twenty years younger, but we are close and mutually supportive. As he is interested in my getting to know better the Afghan interpreters who work with our medical–surgical teams, he organizes a get-together. They host us in their tent, in a very friendly manner, with all of us sitting on the ground around tea and local treats.

One of them, a Tadjik physician, fought the Russian forces under the command of Ahmad Shah Massoud, a friend of the French, who was, perhaps not coincidentally, assassinated two days before 9/11. Almost sixty, tall and skinny, his beard and hair nearly white, this doctor has in his eyes the depth of the warrior who has fought for causes he deemed just. His English is correct. He knows Paris, which he once visited before the Soviet–Afghan war, and has only good things to say about France. I remain prudent, although he seems to believe what he says. He certainly isn't a friend of the Taliban and is, in fact, risking his life by working as an interpreter for NATO forces, but one also has to take the facts into account: in this war of occupation, in which we are seen as crusaders in Muslim territory, our relationships can only be superficial. Moreover, I haven't used my real name in introducing myself in order to avoid evoking my Jewish origins, which can only trigger prejudice in this country. I've heard that one of the last remaining Jews in the area died recently. He lived in Kabul where he took care of the old synagogue.

What will become of these interpreters at the end of this war? They are traitors in the eyes of the insurgents. The British military leadership says they will be protected in exchange for services rendered and accepted, along with their families, in the United Kingdom. Should one believe that? In any case, that would be the best scenario for them, for their lives and those of their families will be worth little if they stay here.

~

One evening, after work, I'm back in my room talking to Bob.

"You've almost reached the end of your mission, Elie," he says. "What do you think of Camp Bastion?"

"I think I could have found a better spot for my vacation, Bob. Like the beach at Saint-Tropez!"

"I've told the entire team that my strange Frenchie roommate wakes up every morning by doing upside-down yoga poses!"

"Of course your English pals would find that funny. You should talk, Bob, you're the one who gets up at five to go jogging!"

"Hey, thanks for 'Hallelujah,'" he says, referring to a version by Jeff Buckley that I gave him on a USB key. "What a great recording!"

"I told you it was. It's very different from the original version sung by Leonard Cohen. You want to hear Eva Cassidy's version of 'Over the Rainbow'?" I ask. "Do you know her? She's an American singer who died too young from skin cancer, but left a few songs that are real gems. You can tell me what you think. . . ."

"Speaking of Americans, have they invited you over there to lunch yet?" he asks, referring to Camp Leatherneck, next door to us.

"Yes, and I saw they have it as good here as they do at Djibouti—huge amounts of food and sweets, especially ice cream. I'm not surprised that some of their soldiers are borderline obese. Not advisable in this climate. . . ."

"Why are the French always anti-American?"

"I'm not anti-American, Bob!" I object. "When I was growing up, everyone around me loved America for liberating us from the Nazis and defeating them. Of course, eventually I came to understand that there was a certain amount of mythology in all of that, and my enthusiasm was moderated a bit. But I still support the US. Better them leading the world than the Russians or Chinese. And I've always had a passion for jazz, which is a product a hundred percent made in USA!"

"I get it."

"And what about your wife, Bob? How's she doing?" I ask. They are about to have their first child.

"Shirley's doing fine. She's in her twenty-eighth week now. For the moment, all is well!"

"You still don't want to know whether it's a boy or a girl?"

"No, let Nature surprise us. I'll be home in time for the delivery. In the end, I'll have been gone for a third of her pregnancy. I miss her, you know. With thirty-five hundred miles between us, I realize how attached I am to her!"

As he talks, I think about Clara and Paul and how much I'm missing them.

"I'm on duty tonight," I say. "What are you going to do with your time off?"

"First I'm going to Skype with my beloved. Then I'll watch a movie on my laptop."

"Lucky dog! I haven't had the time to watch a single one since I got here."

~

The next afternoon, we are transferring two young wounded Afghans to the hospital in Lashkar Gah. They stumbled right into some fighting on leaving their village and have suffered gunshot wounds. They are now convalescing.

Unlike the primary transfers carried out by the MERT, these secondary transfers transport patients whose condition is no longer life-threatening. Either they finish convalescing elsewhere or they require specialized care that isn't available at Camp Bastion, such as neurosurgery or ophthalmology, located at the American hospital in Kandahar. Today Andrew and Natasha are working with me. He's a paramedic and she's a nurse, both recently arrived from England. He has already served in Iraq. For Natasha, it's her first experience in a war zone. Since security is of paramount importance, we have to wait an hour before getting authorization to leave. The risk of an attack continues. I sense our two young Afghan patients would like to communicate with us, to thank us for having taken care of them, but they don't speak English. We can only exchange smiles and kind glances with them.

The flight over the Helmand desert is fascinating. We fly rather low. During the transport, I study the landscape through the porthole I'm sitting next to. It's almost 1:00 p.m. and the light is very strong.

We left Camp Bastion twenty minutes ago. Beneath the intense sun, the sand and loose stones stand out sharply against the blue sky. Suddenly, like a mirage, the Helmand River appears, springing out of nowhere. It's the river that irrigates the Green Zone and its immense fields of poppy flowers, which spread as far as the eye can see toward Pakistan and Iran. The contrast is striking. The green of the crops has suddenly taken the place of the faded yellow of the desert. Helmand is a high-intensity combat zone. The majority of Afghan opium comes from flowers grown here. The main source of revenue for farmers and warlords, it also serves to finance the purchase of arms necessary for this war.

Afghanistan remains the biggest producer of heroin in the world. The Afghan people, including its fighters, consume it, and perhaps also some NATO soldiers. Difficult to ignore if you want to be accepted by the population that lives off it. At the same time, it's necessary to counter the drug cartels and arms traffickers. How is one to undo the strong ties that exist between the farmers and traffickers without eliminating their raw material, opium?

The same problem exists with cocaine in South America. It's the serpent biting its own tail. What would happen to the world economy if it were devoid of its trafficking of drugs, arms, organs, and children, not to mention slavery and prostitution? Are the big banks willing to do without this money that has permeated their system and the offshores?

In this global war, the white-collared mafias seem to have infiltrated the states. All the countries involved are implicated. A big game of chess, where there's no limit to corruption. Terrorism is one of its facets. Are the Americans able or willing to resolve this problem, when the military-industrial lobby is playing an important role in the maintenance of their hegemony? They aren't the only ones, other countries are profiting as well. . . . The answers are blowing in the wind.

15.
THE YOUNG BRITISH SOLDIER

My **mission will** soon be over. After weeks spent in the middle of war, the return to the daily routines of Parisian life will surely seem bizarre. In the late afternoon I've taken advantage of an intermission to go relax at the camp's Starbucks café, a privilege I haven't had the chance to enjoy much since my arrival. Maybe I'm taking a break there now because I finally feel I've finished the job I came to do.

Inside the café, if it weren't for the uniforms, you could think you were in London. Many of these British fighters are the same age as my son, Paul. There he is, a student back in Europe, while these guys here are fighting along a virtual red line separating two civilizations. The same generation, but different destinies. Sipping my cappuccino, I think back over a recent drama I witnessed at Camp Bastion. This episode, representative of the world of communications we now inhabit, plunged me directly into the universe of modern war.

A young British soldier is expected to arrive at the emergency services. As usual, the team is on a war footing. Everything is ready to receive him. When he arrives, we understand quickly that his chances of survival are minimal. Hit in the head by a grenade thrown at the checkpoint he was in charge of, he is now in a coma. His helmet didn't succeed in protecting him. His face is bloodied and swollen, deformed by the trauma. A compression bandage is on his scalp. Beneath it, the explosion fractured his skull. The impact has caused a brain hemorrhage and the consequent edema is exerting downward pressure on the brain, which moves down toward the occipital orb. The rest of his body seems intact. The team will do everything possible to save him, but he'll die before he reaches the CT scan.

In accordance with the protocol, when a soldier falls in combat, the internet and telephone satellite links are instantly cut off in Camp Bastion, to enable authorities to announce the death to his family in England before the media get hold of the story. The atmosphere is heavy, in the hospital as well as the camp.

The day after this difficult experience, I'm relaxing in the recreation room during my break. It's ten in the morning. I glance at the television, which is permanently turned on. The *BBC World News* is addressing an internal political matter. Suddenly the program is interrupted, and the photo of a soldier appears on the screen. He has blue eyes and looks like my son. The journalist announces: "J. D. died yesterday at Camp Bastion. He was twenty-four years old. He joins the hundreds of brothers-in-arms who have been killed in combat over the past ten years. His family is devastated. His fiancée is pregnant. They were supposed to get married when he returned from his mission."

I quickly realize that J. D. is the soldier we received the day before in the emergency department. I'm discovering his actual face and identity only today. The man I saw yesterday had a face deformed, destroyed by his injuries. As for his name, in the turmoil I'd forgotten it.

How strange is the modern world with its almost instantaneous communication networks. Time and distance are abolished. I'm learning today from the *BBC World News*, broadcast in London, 3,500 miles from Afghanistan, the identity and appearance of this young fighter, who died right in front of me, yesterday, here at Camp Bastion!

At the end of the day, I attend the prayer service in his memory, before his body is repatriated to the United Kingdom. It is six in the evening. Soon it'll be dusk, because night falls fast at this latitude. At sunset, the still blue sky is streaked with red. The desert then bathes in a faded light that's very particular and unforgettable. It's hot. Standing in line, at attention, in uniform and with red or green berets, are representatives from all the British units based at Camp Bastion, and almost the entire health service with the exception of those on duty. A Frenchman, I become one with them. It doesn't matter that I'm wearing a different uniform. We are all of us, brothers-in-arms serving the same cause, there in memory of J.D.

The eulogy is poignant. His unit commander and one of his fellow fighters take turns speaking and, with much emotion in their voices, recall J.D. His courage, his sense of friendship, and also his humor. The Anglican priest goes on to give a short sermon giving the basic facts, then concludes with the usual prayers. The ceremony ends with the traditional taps played for the dead and cannon fire. We separate in silence to return to our different activities.

In the meantime, night has fallen. The desert engulfs us again. While I head toward the hospital, my paternal grandfather accompanies me quietly as though he were watching me live these events and grow through them. How is it that I feel his presence so strongly, when I have no memory of him and he died so long ago? The nature and immateriality of this dialogue between our souls goes beyond usual thinking. This mysterious form of energy fascinates me. Perhaps there are other dimensions accessible to us during and after our lifetime.

As for horrors, grandfather Elie certainly saw a lot of them in 1916 at Verdun. The battle lasted nine months and killed 300,000 French and German soldiers altogether. That's not counting the wounded. I can only imagine the long waits in the cold and the mud of the trenches before the murderous attacks. The alcohol needed to handle anxiety. The smell of dead flesh coming from the piles of cadavers lying about, without prayers to accompany them. The wooden crosses improvised for those who were buried too fast. There were twenty million victims in the Great War, mostly soldiers. World War II killed approximately seventy million, including many civilians. This is without counting the wounded, the disabled, and the PTSD cases.

Fortunately what I'm living through at Camp Bastion isn't comparable! With Hiroshima and Nagasaki, the atomic era has modified the situation. The nature and form of conflicts have progressively changed. Using dissuasion as their doctrine, the great powers confronted each other during the Cold War through intermediary countries. The wars in Korea, Indochina, Algeria, and Vietnam are examples. Western thinking has evolved so that public opinion is no longer ready to support war. How long will that last?

At present, confrontation continues, but terrorism has complicated the situation. Religious fanaticism is part of the brew. It's the new ideology. The enemy is not always visible. Guerilla and counterinsurgency scenarios have replaced classic battles between nations of equal military force.

In Afghanistan, the battle is asymmetrical. An over-equipped NATO fights against insurgents armed with machine guns. The enemy advances wearing masks and knowing his terrain perfectly.

He is hard to recognize. The local farmer, who seems quiet and inoffensive, can, for a price, turn into a dangerous warrior, and then return to his field as though nothing had happened.

For these reasons, war has become secret. Fewer famous reporters are penetrating sensitive zones. Televisions are broadcasting images that armies have filmed and chosen for them.

Strategy and tactics are priorities based on intelligence and the use of hyper-trained Special Forces deployed in small numbers. These commandos are more and more computerized, and can access information or transmit it in real time back to headquarters. This increases the precision and speed of their interventions, essential for the success of their missions.

Emphasis is also placed on prevention. A fighter's life is precious. It has been a long time since senile generals sent their troops into slaughter without considering the extent of losses. Today, in contrast, the concept of "zero deaths" has taken hold. On the Afghan terrain, in twelve years, the French have lost eighty-nine lives. This same idea applies to the British as well as the Americans. Today, a fighter is no longer anonymous the way he was at the time of the Unknown Soldier. When he dies, he is celebrated at the highest state level with much pomp and in the media. Even if all this is colored by political demagoguery, one shouldn't complain about it. A soldier deserves his honors.

Modern technology has evolved in this direction, enabling us to perform certain tasks that used to involve the exposure of human beings. War has become cybernetic. The use of drones is one example. In a bunker somewhere in the US, military computer scientists, who become airplane pilots via an interposed monitor screen, can bomb targets thousands of miles away. In the future, robots will be used more and more in theaters of operation.

This new manner of fighting, in which commitment and

risk-taking become nonexistent, can, however, pose ethical problems. The confrontation is almost like a video game, with the difference that humans will die at the other end of the war chain. The result: local populations are affected on a massive scale. Hundreds of thousands of victims during the second Iraq War are evidence that the relationship between military and civilian losses has been inverted, unfortunately for the latter.

This phenomenon isn't new, however. During the Spanish Civil War and World War II, populations often suffered more than soldiers. The Holocaust is a sad and cynical example of this. In different ways, the Russian front and the bombing of French, English, and German cities have also illustrated civilian suffering.

Today, the frontier between the real and virtual worlds is often vague, as the two influence each other. In this process, the role of the hero stands out. My generation identified with Hollywood stars. My son's generation, more digitally connected, finds itself in the middle of video games where it can identify with the fictional hero. This new, disturbed relationship to reality can explain certain personality disorders that are being seen these days.

When I've moved through the Afghan sky by helicopter or airplane, I've sometimes felt myself at the border between dream and reality. Maybe because these scenes resemble those in war movies or older stories that filled my imagination growing up. Against all expectation, this déjà-vu has helped me tolerate the difficulties of the situations I've experienced, because the environment strikes me—incorrectly—as familiar.

But nothing can keep real life from catching up to you. In spite of all the precautions taken, there is no such thing as zero risk.

War is never clean, the way some Americans would like us to believe. It always generates dead and wounded. Those who live through it remain profoundly marked at different levels. Ironically, modern diplomacy talks about maintaining peace. Could it be that it's a hypocritical way of justifying these interventions, faced with reticent public opinion?

16.
KABUL

September 2011. Tomorrow, I'm leaving Camp Bastion to join the French forces at KAIA, the international airport in Kabul. They are expecting me at Kandahar where I must stop on the way.

Harry seems pleased with me when we say goodbye in his office at the hospital. "You've completed your mission, Elie, all the teams are satisfied. The French sent the right person to the right place at the right time!"

"Thanks, but I'm not through with everything yet. I still have to get back to Paris safe and sound and finish writing my report."

"That's right! It'll also be in English, I suppose?"

"Yes! As a first step, I'll turn it into D__, my liaison officer with the British. Then if everything is in order, I'll translate it into French before submitting it to the French."

"So you still have other fish to fry!"

"I know."

~

I'm off duty in order to get ready to leave. I do the laundry quickly, and I'm soon packing my bag. Soldiers need to travel lightly, and I realize with satisfaction that when I packed for this mission, I came with only what was strictly necessary.

Remembering the unpleasant complications involved in my arrival, I've called the French military staff in Kandahar and Kabul in order to confirm the arrangements for my return to France.

"They'll be expecting you in Kandahar tomorrow, in the late morning. A nurse will pick you up at the airport."

"And my flight to Kabul, Colonel?"

"It'll be the day after, in the afternoon. Headquarters have been informed," he says.

After thanking them for their competence, I say goodbye to the teams at Role 3 Hospital, then pass the evening with Bob and his colleagues at the camp pub, drinking nonalcoholic beers and Coca-Cola, talking about this and that one last time.

"When are you going back to London, Bob?"

"End of October. I'll have a three-week vacation in the sun with my wife, then go back to my job as internist at the hospital in November. When will you be in England again?"

"I'll certainly have the opportunity to go back several times between now and the end of the year, because I have to have my report validated by the British."

"Call me when you get there. You can come have dinner with us. I'll introduce you to Shirley, and you can see the baby."

"You bet. In the meantime, take care."

"Have a good trip back to France, Elie."

The morning I leave, riding in the Jeep taking me to the military airport, I have a surreal mixed feeling of attachment to the camp and relief I'm finally leaving it.

The plane is delayed, probably for security reasons. Once we've gone through the check, there are four of us waiting. The atmosphere doesn't lend itself to communication. Each of us is in his or her own bubble, focused on what lies ahead. Besides, there isn't much conversation in these military places, unless you're with colleagues from your unit or buddies. You need to know how to hold your tongue. As I observe them, I realize that, like me, they have specific goals on their minds.

I go over this adventure in my mind. The risks taken and still to be taken. My family, my friends. Time is moving slowly. When you're deep in this universe, you don't know when you'll get out. And if you get to go home, you hope it'll be in good health. Intensifying the sense of being in an interminable tunnel and the attendant anxiety is that fact that the return trip can sometimes be delayed by several weeks because of unpredictable factors related to the war. I know my mission will only be completed when I've stepped onto European soil and handed my report in to the French Army.

~

It's 4:00 p.m. in Kandahar. The flight has lasted less than an hour. There were so few of us on the plane that the Hercules seemed like an enormous, cavernous space.

A French military nurse is waiting for me when I leave the plane. "Hello, Doctor. My name is Fanny, and I've been asked to take you to our unit."

"Do you work in the infirmary I visited before?"

"Yes, I do. The physician colleague you met told us about you. You were lucky to get to go to Camp Bastion. What a great mission!"

"You think so? A little risky, no?"

"Maybe, but compared to mine, yours must have been intense. Not much is happening here, one day is pretty much like another. We're a small unit, our zone is secured, and our activities are

restricted to general medicine. When I signed up, I thought I'd be
doing a lot more than that in Afghanistan."

"I understand. We aren't exposed in the same way in war zones.
I'm an outsider, but they entrusted me with this delicate mission."

"I'm sure that more than one career army doc would like to
have been in your shoes."

A little later, I'm talking to a colonel in the French Air Force.
"Hello, Doc. So, mission accomplished and a safe and sound
return home! Could you ask for anything more?" he says, smiling.

"Yes—to get back to Paris in one piece, Colonel!"

"As for that, it'll happen soon. We've already reserved a seat for
your return flight."

"It's funny, the closer I get to the end, the slower time moves,
and my stay feels interminable. I hope our plane leaves at the
scheduled time. It could be delayed by several days, or even
weeks."

"That would surprise me. You'll be traveling with some bigwigs
and VIPS from the French Army. I think there'll even be a general
in the group. They don't postpone flights of that kind."

"May the angels agree with you, Colonel!" I say.

"How was Camp Bastion?"

"A difficult experience—and out of the ordinary!"

"The officer in charge at the DPSD wants to see you. Tomorrow
you'll be leaving to join French Army headquarters in Kabul."

"This time they're expecting me, I hope?"

"Enough with the teasing, Doc!"

I then go to the camp bar where I find the officer from the
DPSD. "I heard your mission went well," he said.

"You've heard correctly, I see you aren't working in intelligence
for nothing!" I joke with him. "In fact, I think it went very well.
The British seem satisfied. And for me, it was a great learning
experience. I'll write up a complete report for the army."

"Is your morale good? Nothing special you need to flag for us? You were supposed to circulate a bit everywhere?"

"It wasn't easy. I was the only French guy in this sea of British and American personnel. But they let me do a lot of things and seemed happy with my work. As this was a political mission, they calculated and limited the risks I'd be taking to make sure I'd return alive, in spite of the danger. In terms of morale, I'm good. I have the feeling of a job well done."

"Well done indeed! Thank you for your cooperation."

The rest of the day goes by fast. After turning in my weapon, I rest a little, then stroll through the immense recreational area located near the French camp. There, soldiers of all nationalities are sitting at café tables, or doing sports, or browsing in the surplus stores. Much to my surprise, I see, in the middle of the desert, an ice hockey rink where Canadian and American teams are playing against each other. Decidedly, the Yankees don't stint on anything!

Kandahar seems as big as Camp Bastion. In the evening, I visit the American hospital, undoubtedly the most modern facility in Afghanistan, before going to eat in the cafeteria, a real international crossroads where soldiers from various NATO countries meet and eat together.

The next day, the plane that takes me to Kabul is also a Hercules, like the one I took to Kandahar. I am with some British soldiers and Belgian Special Forces. The latter are in charge of security at KAIA International Airport, which is also the location of NATO's Kabul headquarters and of the international hospital run by the French colleagues I'm meeting.

As usual, we take off almost vertically for security reasons. By now I'm familiar with these procedures, developed for the war environment I've been immersed in. At the end of the day, I became a soldier in spite of myself.

~

Our vehicle has now come to a halt on the runway at Bagram military airport. Exposed and dangerous, it orchestrates traffic that is among the most intense in the world. We wait for the green light to leave. It's late afternoon in September, and night is already falling in the middle of Central Asia.

Once again, I wonder if what I've experienced for the past two months is real. Although recently I've felt myself less in communication with my grandfather, Elie, I still feel his presence. As my parents know nothing of my mission, he is the link connecting me to my roots. It supports me.

Finally, we take off once more. The inside of the cabin is dark and hot. As in my other trips, I find a prevailing atmosphere of silence and concentration mixed in with fatigue.

We are always conscious of permanent danger. Recently, an American helicopter was shot down in flight. It was transporting around thirty soldiers from the Special Forces.

~

It's 7:00 p.m. It's night, and I find myself alone with my gear at the KAIA military airport in Kabul. I landed twenty minutes ago, and nobody's there to greet me. The soldiers who traveled with me have all returned to their units. Once again, this damned French "organization"! The flight was delayed for security reasons, but they could have inquired about it.

Luckily, there's an office open in the waiting room, which is otherwise deserted. I head toward an American woman in uniform sitting behind the counter. She's friendly and ready to help.

"Hello, I'm a doctor. I've come from Camp Bastion to join up with my French colleagues. They were supposed to come get me, but there's no one. Could I use your telephone to call the hospital?"

"No problem, Doc!"

I land on the medical director. "Hello, so you've forgotten about me?"

"You're here? We thought the flight had been canceled. Don't budge, we'll send a noncom over there straight away. Sorry."

While waiting, I reflect that my return trip is bizarrely like my arrival. How can they leave me on my own, without a weapon, in an environment that could become dangerous at any moment? The British didn't do that. I smile thinking back on what one of my friends used to say, "France—it's always shit, but once you know that, you can make your peace with it."

During World War II, that friend had been in the evacuation from Dunkirk, days of hell and intense bombing, and then the Resistance. I suppose he knew what he was talking about. He later became a great criminal lawyer.

Finally, my driver arrives and takes me to the cafeteria. There, the French medical team is expecting me for dinner.

The hospital director is a surgeon colonel. It's his first experience in a theater of operations. "You requested to visit KAIA hospital in order to study the way we work, Elie?"

"Yes, Colonel, in the context of the report I'm writing about the British troops, I'd like to have a point of view that includes the two systems."

"We are surely different," he says, "although we also have much experience in war medicine. Don't forget Larrey."

The colonel is referring to Dominique Jean Larrey, a French surgeon in Napoleon's army, and the first doctor to create military pre-hospital rescue teams. Before him, the wounded were left to die on the battlefield. Larrey initiated a tradition of exceptional military medicine that continues in France to this day. He was in some ways the ancestor of civilian emergency services like the SAMU.

"In fact, I'm trying to put into perspective what's positive on either side of the Channel."

"There's surely less activity here than at Camp Bastion. You were in a zone where the fighting was intense, with a lot of poly-traumatized cases."

"That's right."

"We take care not only of French and NATO military, but also of the local population, within the framework of agreements made with the authorities. It's a form of cooperation with this country we're squatting in."

"War also involves political transactions."

"France has a long tradition of colonial and tropical medicine and has always seen to the health of the locals."

"I noticed that happening, to a certain degree, in Djibouti."

"The hospital was built by NATO, but it's the French Army's health service that runs it. The structure is smaller than the one at Camp Bastion, but offers the same technical means, twenty-four hours a day, with the addition of a neurosurgeon and an ophthal-mologist. We also do a lot of internal and general medicine. How long will you be staying with us, Elie?"

"Two days. I'm going back to France in a week. I'll spend my last five days in Warehouse, the headquarters for the French troops."

"Could you give us a talk about Camp Bastion before you leave?"

"Sure thing, Colonel."

∼

In Afghanistan, ISAF, the International Security Assistance Force, is constituted by over 130,000 soldiers coming from forty-eight nations. Theoretically, its role is to counter the Taliban, protect the Afghan people, provide reinforcements for the Afghan security forces, and support their autonomy, as well as to help the Afghan government and support the economic development of the country. In reality, they lack the capacity to fulfill all those functions and are often impeded by local corruption.

There are several other base camps around KAIA headquarters at the Kabul international airport. KAIA is located ten miles from the center of the capital, surrounded by mountains. We are moving toward mid-September and here, in the northern part of the country, autumn has already begun.

I feel the difference in temperature. It is markedly less hot than it was in the Helmand Desert. My uniform is more suitable to this environment than to the one at Camp Bastion. It is finally coming in handy at the end of my mission.

Here, as everywhere in Afghanistan, security is a major issue. In spite of continual surveillance performed by the Belgian Special Forces, a maintenance worker can get caught in an explosion at any time, or a commando of military insurgents in disguise can penetrate the interior of the camp and fire on anything that moves before being itself shot down.

The mission of the American, British, and French forces is to train the Afghan Army, and there are inevitably serious problems that arise in the process. Last week, American troops were killed without warning by an Afghan soldier who turned against them. As in Kandahar and Camp Bastion, there's the risk that rockets launched from outside will land by chance on buildings or on us. All movement outside the camp involves armed soldiers in armored vehicles. And then there are the unavoidable checkpoints and their searches.

In this horizontal, prefabricated Tower of Babel, 4,000 people from different countries work side by side without really talking to each other. Many of them circulate with their weapons, constantly ready to retaliate. This in itself can create problems, as shots can be fired accidentally. Communication is impeded by the secrecy of the operations, for a mission's success requires a certain reserve. Information is released in bits and pieces, except at the highest level of command. Even there, I imagine that the American military command filters the messages it shares with its allies.

KAIA isn't as big as Kandahar or Camp Bastion, but it boasts a high-tech sports facility, bars where you can order nonalcoholic drinks, and a cafeteria located in a space that looks like a big gymnasium decorated with the flags of the fifty allied nations. Everyone there eats with his hand on the trigger. The slightest incident, like the false rumor of an attack can lead to a round of deadly shooting!

There is even a little market, a kind of bazaar, where authorized Afghans sell traditional clothing, carpets, and precious stones. In Central Asia as elsewhere in Asia, bargaining is the rule, and you can acquire an emerald or a lapis lazuli at a reasonable price. As in France under German occupation during World War II, some Afghans have built up fortunes by collaborating with the American forces. There will certainly be accounts to settle after the allies leave.

Last night, toward two in the morning, there was an earthquake. The shaking lasted a few seconds, just long enough to wake me up. I thought it was an explosion, and then I went back to sleep. It's at breakfast I heard the news. There wasn't too much damage. Mini earthquakes often happen in this part of the world, which is sensitive to the movement of tectonic plates.

This afternoon, I went to the headquarters of the French Forces at Camp Warehouse, after having crossed part of Kabul and its periphery in an armored vehicle. It's a metropolis marked by war. The roads are in poor condition.

Through the tinted windows, under the sun, I can see the dilapidated buildings and the shantytowns alongside the occasional official building and the luxurious villas belonging to drug traffickers. Since my arrival in this theater of operations, I've spent my time in military camps, airplanes, and helicopters, and now I have for the first time the furtive impression of being immersed in the daily life of this country. But it's only an illusion. We are armed to the teeth, ready to use our weapons at any moment.

Our chauffeur is under orders to drive at a regular speed without stopping. You have to be on your guard because the smallest traffic jam can turn into a trap. People here drive without licenses. The cars and two-wheeled vehicles going by in the dust swirling up from the beaten earth are often half-busted. There are no road signs or traffic lights, and it's easy for someone coming in the opposite direction to crash into you.

I don't see a single Afghan woman on the way. They stay at home. I've hardly seen any Afghan women during my mission, except one time, at the hospital in Kabul, a mother who was accompanying her sick child. Some men are in traditional dress with a *pakol* on their heads, the flat beret in felted beige wool made famous by Massoud. Others wear jeans and long-sleeved shirts. They are not supposed to show any part of their body.

My impression is one of general poverty in this underdeveloped country where illiteracy and unemployment rule. Thirty years of conflict haven't improved matters any.

∼

Camp Warehouse is situated near KAIA. It's run by the Turkish Army. Turkey plays a limited role in this war. Its 1,800 soldiers engaged on the ground do not take part in combat. In order to satisfy the demands of their Muslim brothers, they limit their activities to the training of Afghan security forces and to reconstruction projects.

The atmosphere is calm. The war seems far away. However, I

remain vigilant. I have no weapon with me. I am unnerved by the idea that I cannot defend myself in the event of danger.

If all goes well, my plane should leave in five days. On my return, I won't stop in Cyprus to decompress with the other soldiers. Doing that would, however, be a good idea. After doing their duty, the French and British units usually spend three days there. Relaxation, big hotels at the seaside, massages, saunas, cultural visits, and psychological evaluations for PTSD are all on the agenda.

It can be difficult for fighting personnel to return to ordinary life after six months of intensive service. The mental health teams have to help them deactivate mental mechanisms honed for combat. They also help soldiers regulate stress and detect which ones are having problems. Armies are today very aware of post-combat emotional trauma. The veterans of the Great War weren't as fortunate. Many of them ended up in mental asylums after the fighting ended.

As for me, as soon as I get back, I will return to my work at the SAMU. So I might as well try to enjoy this down time at Warehouse.

The hours pass slowly, as though measured out slowly with a dropper, undoubtedly because, after what I've been through, I'm not used to having nothing to do. They're putting me up with officers and noncoms, I have a room that looks out over a lovely patio.

At noon, in the cafeteria, I run into the minister whom I'd met in Kandahar before leaving for Camp Bastion. "Your mission has been difficult, Elie. You managed well for a supposed amateur. The first time I saw you, I understood you were a being of light."

"Don't you think you're exaggerating a bit, Reverend?"

"When I appreciate someone, it's a hundred percent. Sorry, but that's the verdict!"

"Yeah, okay, let's say you're also here to help me release my stress, like the psychiatrist I met in Kabul, whom I ended up liking a lot. I'm lucky running into you. I could use a metaphysical conversation to get me through this hostile environment."

"You're on! I'm your man!"

"Have you had the opportunity to go to advanced positions in Kapisa?" I ask, referring to a province in the northeast of the country.

"Yes, periodically."

"Do soldiers talk to you about their struggle to find meaning in this war, about handicap and death?"

"They do. About their family relationships, too, when they're far from those they love for months at a time."

"Do you believe couples can remain faithful during these periods of long separation?"

"They're men and women, not angels, and the flesh remains weak."

"Does that maxim apply to ministers as well?" I ask, daringly.

"The minister is also a human being, and even if he is married, he can also have a moment of weakness, but not while on a foreign operation. Here I have to set a good example, and I'm determined to do the job well. You can't fool around during times of war!"

"You were just speaking about beings of light. It seems that last week, Neil Armstrong came to KAIA to speak to American troops and raise their morale."

"That's right, Elie. I went to hear him talk. It was fantastic!"

"I imagine it was luminous, no? What a mythical figure . . . It's too bad, I missed seeing him by just a few days."

"But at least you can say you were in the country at the same time!"

"A nice way to reframe it, Reverend!"

∽

That afternoon, I meet with the head of the French intelligence services in Afghanistan. During a conversation that lasts over two hours, we talk about my mission and the strange events that brought me here. Like Bob, he speaks to me as a brother-in-arms.

"In reality, you didn't have an obligation to serve," he says, "but you did."

"What do you mean?"

"You thought you had a debt. Maybe, but not the one you think. The problem of your military dossier being at the General Medical Council could have been resolved some other way. You're not the only one who did stupid things in his youth."

"And the Israelis in all this?"

"Logical! You're Jewish, your profile interested them. They tried to recruit you, it didn't work out, that's all there is to it."

"Do you think they were from the Mossad?"

"Hard to say, because Israeli intelligence is huge. Their contacting you was probably sponsored by them, but by which branch exactly, I don't know."

"And was that girl, Laura, mixed up in any of this?"

"We don't seem to have anything on her. Maybe she was in contact with them, and now she's a sleeper agent. Whatever the case, be careful when you see her again."

"I'm not planning on it; I've cut off all communication with her! You sure you're telling me the whole truth?"

"You know a bit about how our services function. For security reasons, we're only giving you the information that you need at the moment. . . ."

"I'm left wondering why I came and what this was all about."

"It was meant to be, Elie. Tomorrow you return to France. Your return flight has been confirmed. The plane will leave from KAIA."

After all is said and done, I remain in the dark about the forces acting upon my destiny.

17.
RETURNING TO PARIS

September 2011. The French Air Force is taking us back to Paris. The plane took off from KAIA airport in the late morning. Inside, soldiers are going home after six months' absence. Before boarding, they give me the NATO medal for services rendered. I wasn't expecting it. I've never chased after decorations. In the end, I'm simply thankful and happy to be safe and sound. Thanks to Providence.

Through the window, against the blue Afghan sky, I see desert mountain landscapes, emerald lakes and, in the distance, over the foothills of the Himalayas, the eternal snows of the mythical Hindu Kush.

Once again, I realize that I've seen only the dark side of this magical country, the struggles of war, the blood of the wounded, the sound of military planes and helicopters, and the camps filled with soldiers from all over the world. The only Afghans I've met are wounded Taliban prisoners and a few civilians, including children who'd played with IEDs.

I have the feeling of having bypassed this land full of mystery and contrasts. It's hard to believe that Muslims, Buddhists, Christians, and Jews lived here together for centuries. I picture the caravans traveling toward China, along the Silk Road, although I know that what I am imagining is only a stereotype, because invasions and wars have often marked the history of this part of the world.

In spite of everything, I have been able to grasp certain geopolitical realities hidden behind the opaque screens masking the reasons for this American war. However, I've only had access to a fraction of the truth. From here on in, my take on world events and media commentary will be different.

News about current wars, broadcast by television, is often filmed by the audiovisual services of the various armies. For security reasons, it's not a good idea to reveal everything. The reality on the ground is very different from what professional politicians and reporters tell us. And then there is corruption. Whence comes the prevalent confusion. I go home even more aware of the complexity of our little planet.

If all goes well, we should land at Roissy tomorrow toward three in the morning after a stop at Abu Dhabi, then another in Cyprus. During the trip, the plane will fly through Pakistan's air space. We need to have that country's permission to continue the flight, otherwise—return to Kabul. The ordeal isn't over yet.

I think about my family. I'm looking forward to seeing everyone. I've exchanged emails with Paul and Clara, who are waiting for me. They have supported me a lot, and I've missed them. Paul has demonstrated great maturity in managing his anxiety about my situation. I also know that Clara and I will be turning over a new leaf.

My parents still don't know about my return. I wanted to surprise them, but news from home led me to change my plans.

Before taking off from Kabul, I turned my cell back on. There was in my voice mail a message from my father, announcing that my mother's older sister has died. The burial is scheduled for the day after I land.

In an uncanny sequence of events, it happens that, right when I see the message, I'm getting ready to reread a poetic short story written by Maurice, the son of this deceased aunt. The title is, "A Nail Doesn't Make Blood Gush as Fast as an Insult." I've brought it with me for no clear reason. A subtle combination of science fiction and metaphysics, this narrative speaks of destiny and parallel worlds. Coincidence or synchronicity, the first time I saw my cousin Maurice, he was coming back from another war. The Algerian war. Later on, he would become my first hero and be my mentor during my rebellious adolescence. A solitary being, he was cut down in the fullness of youth by an incurable cancer. At that time, I was a medical student, and Maurice's early death made me understand the limitations of my future profession.

Decidedly, destiny has thick skin and still goes on unfurling its story. A long cycle is being completed. Memories of dear relatives, now gone, continue to appear. After my grandfather, there was my cousin. My memory of him unfolds subtly, like Ariadne's thread, and helps me understand what is happening to me. The quest for the self on the Silk Road . . . At present, I'm convinced that the departed help us in difficult moments. I like the idea of these invisible and intricate ties, woven forever.

The Pakistani authorities have finally authorized our plane to fly over their territory. So much the better, we will finally be leaving the war environment. The return trajectory is open. I will leave a little of myself in this part of the world. And I'll need a lot of time to process this story.

Abu Dhabi. Our first stop. It recently became a French military base. The Foreign Legion has recently left Djibouti in order to move here.[2] We are confined to the airport, situated in the desert in the middle of nowhere. The group is silent. The fatigue is palpable. We have all been marked by our stay in Afghanistan. The American F16s that take off against the setting sun remind us that the war isn't far away. I take advantage of the stop to call my parents. In summer French time is two hours earlier than Abu Dhabi.

"Where are you, Elie?"

"I'm in London, Dad."

"Did you get my message about your aunt?"

"Yes, I'm coming home this evening. I'll come to the burial."

They're happy I'll be there tomorrow for the ceremony. All that remains for me to do now is to tell them the truth. We'll see.

Roissy, three o'clock in the morning. After a brief stop in Cyprus where a majority of the troops disembark in order to take three days of leave, the rest of the trip takes place without any problems. Time passes quickly.

The soldiers traveling with me were all expected and have rejoined their respective units. Not knowing exactly when I'd arrive, I told Clara not to come get me, so I need to get back home on my own. At this hour, the local commuter train between the airport and Paris isn't running. There aren't any taxis, either. I am alone, in uniform, my military bag on my back, in the arrival hall of the deserted airport, which is lit up with blue neon lighting. All this seems strange after such an intense experience at the front. This landing back in my life feels raw.

Suddenly, two men come out of nowhere approach me. One of them addresses me.

"Eighty euros to get back to Paris, soldier?"

---

2   The Foreign Legion has since left Abu Dhabi and returned to France. *Note J.L.*

"You're a taxi driver? That's too much! I'll wait for the first train."

The other man butts in, "Forty euros!"

He is wearing a *djellaba*, the long loose robe typically worn in North Africa. Funny outfit for a Parisian taxi driver. I think again about Afghanistan. I hesitate, but still, I want to get home fast.

"Thirty euros! Not more!"

"It's hardly worth my while, but for a French soldier—it's agreed."

"You're joking! The taxi light is off. You were off duty, so it's all profit for you!"

While talking to him, I put my stuff in the trunk after making sure that I've got my switchblade with me. A slightly paranoid reflex on the part of someone returning from war. This guy is shabby but surely less dangerous than a Taliban.

As we head toward Paris, he tries to talk to me several times. He mentions Islam, integration, terrorism, Algeria, the country of his ancestors and dear to his heart. I hear him without really listening. My head is elsewhere. What am I doing in this taxi with this guy in a *djellaba* born in France, who says he doesn't feel French? Westerners are fighting in Muslim lands, 3,400 miles from here, while dishonest and irresponsible politicians would have us believe the war is not the result of a shock of civilizations. We swim in the absurd. It's all Kafkaesque. Has the time of the Crusades returned?

I can't know for sure, but this war without a front could easily arrive in our cities and countrysides if we aren't careful. Today, in what are called zones of lawlessness, thousands of young people are ready to fight against a system that has largely forgotten them. Religious fanaticism seems an answer to their frustrations. Are they aware that this remedy is a poisonous one?

At present the only thing that counts for me is the initiatory experience I've lived through. In developing my intuition, it has also revealed to me my timeless connection with my paternal grandfather. It seems that the traumas of one generation can be passed down to the following ones. During World War I, at Verdun or elsewhere, Elie must have experienced enormous horrors that he said little about to either his wife or children. The culture and thinking of the times were very different. Perhaps it was necessary for someone at the other end of the chain—me, his grandson—to go to war in order to do the work of reparation. He was a fighter, I am a doctor. He certainly took other men's lives, even though he told my father he often fired his rifle in the air. On my end, I tried to care for and heal the wounded. Resilience has no age. It crosses time and space.

EPILOGUE

As this translation goes to press, history is still being written. At the end of 2014, the British Army withdrew from Camp Bastion, the structure of which was almost completely taken apart. Part of it was shipped back to the UK. The remaining part was renamed Camp Shorabak and is now being used by the Afghan Army. The largest British base since World War II is nothing but a shadow of its previous self, a ruin, a mirage in the Helmand desert.

Over the course of fourteen years of war, the British military operation cost 50 million euros, a sum larger than that spent on any other conflict. And this war, the longest in the history of the United States, has not yet wound down.

Between 2001 and 2016, there were, according to available counts, over 110,000 deaths, including 2,371 American soldiers, 454 British soldiers, 89 French soldiers, 675 soldiers from other coalition countries, 30,000 Afghan military and police personnel, 31,000 Afghan civilians, almost 4,000 humanitarian workers, journalists, and contractors, and finally 42,000 Taliban and other insurgents. This doesn't take into account the innumerable wounded, some of them disabled for the rest of their lives.

The Taliban remain on the ground in competition with the Islamic State, opium traffic continues and has even increased, the country remains corrupt, and the condition of women hasn't really changed.

The conflict has spread from Central Asia to Africa, passing through the Middle East. After 9/11 it touched Mumbai, Madrid, London, Brussels, and Paris, impacting civilian populations once again. As if to underscore Europe's failure in this war, terrorist suicide attacks are often perpetrated by young Muslims or Muslim converts who are themselves citizens of the country they are targeting. The possibility of political destabilization and interreligious conflicts continues to exist. No continent has been spared. All this resembles a world war of a third type, for the moment a low-intensity one, a kind of globalized guerilla warfare in which terrorism and religion are only two aspects. Behind the interfaith confrontation between Sunni and Shiite factions, the great powers of the world are pushing their pawns on the big chessboard configured by economics and geopolitics. War is also a business.

As for me, paradoxically this experience strengthened me. It came to feel like the product of destiny, the result of a subtle confluence between circumstances and free will. The head of the French intelligence services in Afghanistan was right when he said that I had a debt to pay, but perhaps not the one I thought. To my grandfather? To the army? My answer continues to change, because I still don't know, but I've accepted not knowing because I learned a lot on both a human and professional level. The main thing is that I know that my experience was useful.

As a consequence of my report, the British and American Damage Control Resuscitation protocols I studied in Afghanistan are now being taught in France, in the university curricula for emergency medicine. When possible, its principles are used to treat victims of terrorist attacks.

If only for that reason, my mission will have made an important contribution. As in France, terrorism can hit populations in cities as well as elsewhere. The health workers of the SAMU and hospital emergency departments are now trained in war medicine and in how to secure hostile zones, because the paradigms of catastrophic medicine have changed. In the current context, there can be no truly secure zones because a first attack can be prelude to a secondary one that happens on the same site while emergency services are arriving. The dramas of *Charlie Hebdo* and the Hyper Casher[3] served as warnings about the multisite operational capabilities of these assailants.

Faced with this situation, pre-hospital health care workers are exposed to danger in a way they never have been before. Those who are connected to the BRI, the RAID, the GIGN[4], and the fire department have chosen the job and are trained for it. But the others, the civilians employees of the SAMU, many of whom have families, have not a priori signed up to work in combat zones. Many of them, and it's understandable, were psychologically impacted by what they experienced on November 13, 2015, during the attacks on the Bataclan Club. Of course, some had undergone training for catastrophic scenarios of this kind, organized regularly by the Paris SAMU. In an ironic twist of fate, a logistical simulation of a multiple-site attack had taken place that same morning, with the

---

3   On January 15, 2015, Paris suffered the first of a cluster of terrorist attacks when the headquarters of the satirical newspaper, *Charlie Hebdo*, was targeted. This was followed two days later by an attack on a kosher supermarket, Hypercasher.

4   BRI stands for Brigade Rapide d'Intervention; RAID for Recherche, Assistance, Intervention, Dissuasion; and GIGN for Groupe d'Intervention de la Gendarmerie Nationale.

fire brigade, the SAMU of the Ile-de-France region, and the rescue workers of the Red Cross and the Protection Civile all participating. But reality always outdoes fiction. Unfortunately, they had their baptism by fire that very night, and they are now conscious of the stakes. So are their supervisors, who have since reflected much on the subject, especially on the technical and psychological preparation needed, as well as on physical protection. (It is worth noting here that there is little insurance for health care workers who are victims of terrorist attacks, which fall in the category of war casualties and are not covered by regular policies.) With the apparent mobilization of political actors, the police and *gendarmerie* have rightfully demanded more means and suitable training programs.

The experience of the army remains of utmost importance in the context of urban guerilla warfare. In a democracy, with the exception of martial law, the management of this kind of crisis remains the prerogative of prefects and police forces. However, soldiers, as well as military doctors and nurses who have been deployed in Afghanistan, Africa, and the Middle East, have the necessary qualities to help train civilian health professionals and assure their protection, if needed. All these institutions must find ways to coordinate their respective roles and activities for the good of the population. Union makes for strength.

Volunteer general practitioners trained for terrorist attacks could reinforce the system. The speed and quality of the care of victims and affected professionals has improved since the Bataclan attack, although the long-term care for resulting psychological trauma, often severe, is not always sufficient.

Connections and exchanges of knowhow among the different European services providing emergency medicine already exist, but need to be developed further. This process, necessarily dependent upon political decision-makers, will require permanent vigilance as well as a willingness to adapt to the evolution of events.

It is worth noting that the Damage Control Resuscitation that I witnessed at Camp Bastion and the procedures applied in urban guerilla warfare differ in some ways. To begin with, soldiers are committed professionals who are aware of the risks they are taking and trained to deal with them. They know that disability or death may wait for them at the end of their mission, and they are expected to accept the consequences. Deployment in a war zone involves an apprenticeship requiring not only motivation, but also self-denial and a readiness for sacrifice which can, in some cases, become extreme. In contrast, even if they are competent and devoted to serving others, health care workers in the civilian world have not been initiated into combat culture, at least not yet.

Finally, civilian victims of attacks are not trained in rescue techniques the way professional fighters on the ground are. Indeed, the average soldier has had some of this training and carries with him an emergency kit containing morphine, a tourniquet, and hemostatic dressings, in order to bring under control hemorrhages resulting from mines and gunfire. Indeed, the key concept of Damage Control Resuscitation is the crucial importance of coming to the rescue of one's fellow fighters, or even oneself, in the first ten to fifteen minutes. This was certainly not what happened at the Bataclan, where victims were stranded without help for at least an hour and a half. As for the second concept of Damage Control Resuscitation, namely massive blood transfusions starting in the combat zone, it is not, at present, implemented in urban areas.

On this subject, it is interesting to observe the way in which the Israelis manage these problems, which they have been facing for decades. Unlike Western countries (except Switzerland), the State of Israel, which has been at war since its creation in 1948, has an army of conscripted soldiers. Military service lasts for two years for women and three for men. As a direct consequence of this policy, most civilians have been trained in rescue techniques, firearms, and security issues. The country is itself set up like a fortress. One thus finds oneself in a military context in which the police and citizens have supporting roles in defense. This picture is closer to what I lived within the military coalition in Afghanistan.

In yet another coincidence, I found myself in Jerusalem in the summer of 2014, right in the middle of the Israel-Gaza conflict. Although I was still under contract with the operational reserve of the French Army, I went there in a private and professional capacity.

During my stay, I had the opportunity to meet one of the founders of Unit 669, an elite corps of the Israeli Air Force that specializes in rescue operations in extreme situations. This doctor and I exchanged stories about our experiences, his in Israel, mine in Afghanistan, which turned out to be not very different, as the Israeli, American, British, and French military health services collaborate regularly.

For me, I came full circle that day in Jerusalem. My adventure, which had begun in London in a misunderstanding with so-called agents of the Mossad, ended with this straightforward, high-level meeting.

Back from Camp Bastion, I had to tell my parents and my sister about my Afghan mission. Once again, coincidence or synchronicity, I did it the morning of my return when I went to the burial of my mother's older sister, the mother of my cousin and mentor, Maurice. As a result, one drama replaced another, and the family ceremony took on another mood, as though my unexpected journey to Afghanistan, by virtue of its exotic and offbeat character, relaxed the heavy atmosphere of the funeral.

I think that no one truly realized at the time what kind of hell I'd returned from and what I'd lived through. Later, my father did experience a certain pride when he saw the medals the army had given me, but in my eyes the Combatant's Cross[5] I received will never have the same value as the Military Cross awarded to my grandfather. As for my war without a front, he was the one who helped me psychologically to wage it. In an episode that intensified this irrational feeling, one of his sons recently showed me his last letter, written a few days before his death. His last words were for me: "Take good care of Elie, my grandson. I love him so much."

I remain convinced that there is a direct connection between World War I and actual events. Since 9/11 and the Iraq War, the Sykes-Picot agreement, which formed the blueprint for the region a century ago, is no longer relevant. Ideologies are required to pit the peoples of different lands against each other. In 1914, nationalism led millions of people to fight for their countries naively, without any idea of the length of the conflict or the amount of suffering that lay ahead. In 1939, Nazism led to a similar cataclysm. These days, religion has become the prime engine of conflicts.

There is something irrational behind the mechanisms driving war, which economic and geopolitical circumstances don't suffice to explain, as though at given moments the destiny of humankind escapes us and is subjected to incontrollable forces that take things to extreme horror.

These days, cyber- and aerospace warfare have replaced my grandfather's war. In the future, if wars continue to exist, robots will fight alongside men who have been "augmented" by nanotechnologies and artificial intelligence. This has already begun with drones and so-called "human enhancement," which modifies the human body in order to optimize its physical performance. Soon, a "brain computer interface" will enable us to improve an individual's emotional and cognitive capacities, with one of the

---

5 *La Croix du combattant* is a French military decoration in existence since 1930.

stated goals being the protection of the soldier and the ability to save his life.

What I saw at Camp Bastion—a true laboratory of war medicine—with regard to the logistics of rescuing fighters, will surely contribute to the evolution of medicine and raise certain ethical questions. In the meantime, ideas about the end of life and handicap continue to evolve and should also be discussed in the military arena. For example, why save everyone no matter what? What is to become of a soldier who has had two legs and an arm amputated and has also lost his testicles? Shouldn't this mutilated human being have a say about the future of his body? Mightn't he formulate advanced directives in which he would refuse to be left in a vegetative state?

On the other hand, advances in medicine may answer some of these questions thanks to mechatronics and genetic therapies. Intelligent prostheses for the limbs already exist and enable remarkable performance in sports. Paraplegics will soon be walking thanks to exoskeletons. The future may have in reserve for us happy surprises in these areas.

Confronted with extreme situations in which death was prowling about at all times, I have become more conscious of the fragility of life and of my own finiteness, and this adventure has paradoxically brought me closer to my fellow men and taught me a deeper compassion for humanity. The blood I saw spilled was the same color for everyone.

I like the idea, circulating now, that long ago the tribes of Israel traveling toward Central Asia may have established themselves in the country of the Pashtuns and mixed with them. Ironically, these Afghan Muslims who have become fanatics may have Jewish roots.

However, if modern jihadism has grown and spread in Afghanistan since the Soviet–Afghan War, one of its ideological sources can be found among the Muslim Brotherhood created during the 1920s in Egypt. (Another source stems from Saudi Wahhabism). During World War II, the Great Mufti of Jerusalem, Al Husseini, the religious and political leader of Palestinian Arabs and close to the Muslim Brotherhood, rallied to Nazism and its monstrosities. Behind all of this lurks the specter of millenarian fanatics of religions of the book, who are obsessed with "the end of time." One of the goals of jihadism is to use terror to destabilize our societies and to drag us into the apocalyptic trap of a war of civilizations, although its first victims are Muslims themselves as well as Christians from the Middle East who have been persecuted by the Islamic State.

Were young French Muslims or converts who joined the ranks of the Islamic State in Syria aware of how they were manipulated? Often frustrated in their daily lives, attracted by the possibility of adventure, they were ready to do battle with our societies, which they see as devoid of ideals. The all-powerfulness of violence and the fascination with death became their last refuge. There is in this a kind of nihilism exploited by pseudo-scholars of the Koran. Wahhabi-Salafism, originally financed by Saudi Arabia, appeals to their anger toward our society and sells them a program they pay for with their lives.

Our Western societies, focused on materialism and individualism, offer nothing that can compete with this kind of totalitarianism and metaphysics of death, whence comes the risk of rising populisms.

So have the Afghanistan and Iraq wars served any purpose?

Are they part of a new Great Game that is being played between the US, Russia, and China to control Central Asia, a game replacing the one that used to exist between the British Empire and the Russian Empire?

The United States is a great democracy that, in order to continue to play its role as leader of the free world, is forced to make
war or maintain peace. It consequently relies on a very powerful
military-industrial lobby. But even if wars are sometimes necessary, there is certainly cause to reflect on the manner in which
they are waged. The counterinsurgency strategy that I witnessed
in Afghanistan has far from achieved its objectives. You can't
impose democracy on a tribal country where corruption rules and
the religion is at the opposite extreme of American culture. The
concept of a so-called "axis of evil" is simplistic, even dangerous.

At present, weapons rule and might makes right. The Americans
have exported their wars. The consequence has been the destabilization of countries where they intervene, but as is customary with
them, it is others who inherit the problems they create and their
collateral effects. I think of the populations of migrants touched by
the wars in Iraq, Syria, and Libya who are surging toward Europe.

In this apparent confusion, terrorism is the tree that hides the
forest. Politicians use the fear of terrorism as an efficient means
of controlling populations by suggesting the existence of a permanent and supposedly unknown enemy ready to kill them. The
threat hangs over everyone like a sword of Damocles.

But war has many causes. When I was a medical student thirty
years ago, my professors were already talking about the need to
fight against the differences between the Northern and Southern
Hemispheres, in order to avoid potential conflicts and massive
migrations of populations. Courses on the environment discussed pollution and climate change as geopolitically destabiliz-
ing influences. In the West, military strategy takes these factors
into account. But what have we done since then to remedy some of
these root causes of war? Not enough.

This war without a front has become a war for each one of us.
Against poverty and ignorance. For education, the protection of

the environment, and health. If humanity can pull through, a new world may come out of this planetary ordeal. If this proves to be the case, human civilization will, after a painful childbirth, no longer be the same. Let us hope its change will be for the better.

Muhammad himself lived near the Jewish communities of Mecca. It is said that he had approximately fifteen wives and concubines, including two Jewish ones, Rayhana and Safiyah, and a Copt Christian one, Maria. The Prophet's genealogical links with Abraham are one of the foundations of Islam, which also recognizes Yeshua, known as Jesus of Nazareth, born of a Jew, and Miriam, who became the Virgin Mary.

Since then, the religions issued from these great figures have not stopped fighting one another. How long this will go on, God only knows . . . In the meantime, everyone wears his cross, his crescent, or his Star of David.

At present, an intellectual current called transhumanism is predicting a radical transformation of humanity. This philosophy takes its inspiration from advances in the augmentation of human intellectual and physical capacities, as well as progress in nanotechnologies, biology, computer science, and neuroscience. But beyond good and evil, the philosophers of transhumanism dream of humans transforming themselves so radically through implants and external devices that they will be "post-human." Immortal, and more. A veritable totalitarian ideology is in the process of being born. Multinational companies are already working on it, the movement has been launched.

Will Augmented Man behave differently?

It's unlikely. This idea of improving the race already existed in the experiments conducted by Dr. Mengele at Auschwitz, the danger being that the bionic man promised for tomorrow might take control over the rest of the human species with a new risk of extermination at the end of it all.

At the end of World War II, the Americans and Russians welcomed Nazi scientists to their countries. The best known of them, Wernher von Braun, the father of the V2 (the first missiles that could have carried atomic weapons), was even one of the administrators at NASA in charge of conquering the moon.

Here on Earth, nothing is completely white or completely dark; the world is rather gray. All this makes me think of the story of the Tower of Babel, an example of human ego pushing to reach the sky.

While waiting for post-human civilization, I will have to be content with simply being a man. That in itself is already not so easy. Stardust, lost in the universe, I look for beauty amid the nonsense. Medical treatments may have become more sophisticated to match humanity's ever-evolving means of destruction, but in spite of all our technological and medical advances, two things have not changed over the centuries: men make war, and we cannot escape the human predicament of having consciousness in bodies destined to suffer. I am reminded of the famous "Ballad of the Hanged Man" by the medieval French poet François Villon, Arthur Rimbaud's virtual brother in poetry. In his poem, Villon spoke compassionately of those whose bodies were decomposing on the gallows. Through them, he gives voice to human fragility:

> *Human brothers, who live on after us,*
> *Let not your hearts be hardened against us,*
> *For if you have pity for us poor ones*
> *God will have that much more for you, thank you*
> *You see us attached here, five, six*
> *As for the flesh we have nourished too much*
> *It has long been devoured and rotten*
> *And we, bones, become ash and powder*
> *No one makes fun of our pain*

But pray that God may absolve us all!
But pray that God. . . .
But pray. . . .
But. . . .
(Trans. J.L.)

GLOSSARY

DPSD: Direction de la Protection et de la Sécurité de la Défense, the French military intelligence service. In October 2016 the name of this organization was changed to DRSD for Direction du Renseignement et de la Sécurité de la Défense.

FOB: Forward Operating Base, a forward position used to support tactical operations. Medical services at a FOB are more limited than the ones at the main bases.

Gendarmerie: There are two police forces in France. The Police Nationale is a civilian one. The Gendarmerie Nationale is part of the French armed forces, working in the civilian context. Its members are military, but they are governed by the Ministry of Interior.

The Great Game: The political confrontation that took place between the British and Russian Empires in Afghanistan between 1830 and 1895.

The Green Zone: A stretch of cultivated land along the Helmand River Valley, in Afghanistan, where poppies are the principal crop. Not to be confused with the Green Zone that was the international zone for the Coalition Provisional Authority in central Baghdad during the American occupation of Iraq after 2003.

IED: Improvised explosive device.

KAIA: Kabul International Airport.

MERT: Medical Emergency Response Team.

Pieds-noirs: French citizens of European descent who were born or lived in Algeria after the French conquest of the territory in 1830 from the Ottoman Empire.

Role 3: In the military, the name of the hospital at any main camp, including Camp Bastion, which is capable of the most advanced care. (Role 1 provides first aid on the field, Role 2 is a light structure close to the field, providing basic surgery.)

SAMU: Service d'Aide Médicale Urgente, the French pre-hospital emergency service available throughout France.

Sykes-Picot: The 1916 agreement that divided spheres of influence between the UK and France in the Middle East. It marks the end of Ottoman influence and power in the region.

Tzahal: The Israeli Defense Force.

ACKNOWLEDGMENTS

would like to thank the following:

My family: Elie, my grandfather. My dear parents, Lucien and Raymonde Cohen, and my sister Danielle. Maurice Bensoussan. Chantal. Hadrien Paul.

My teachers, who have also been my friends: Simone Dy Ruy. Professor Pierre Cornillot. Professor Jean-Claude Legrand. Charley Attali. André Blanc Rosset. Alain Lebret. Audrey Percival Smith. Tosca Marmor. Mahesh.

My friends: Louis Dupin. Menahem Koppleman. Octave Mancuso. Chris Payne. Paul Robertson. Professor Jacques Demongeot. Michel Marlière and his wife Marie-Lise, who encouraged me to write this book. My friend Jean-Pierre Guéno, without whom this project would not have come to term. Rémi Pelletier.

The French and the British military.

Le Passeur Éditeur, for their production of the French edition.

Jessica Levine, for her talent and her excellent translation.

Professor Donald Anderson, for accepting a portion of this manuscript for publication in *War, Literature, and the Arts.*

Brooke Warner, Lauren Wise, and the team at SparkPress, for their superb work.

Caitlin Hamilton Summie and Rick Summie, for their hard work on publicity.

ABOUT THE AUTHOR

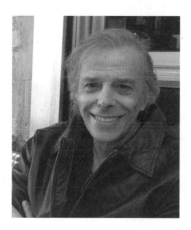

A **pacifist in his youth,** Elie Paul Cohen was a musician before becoming a doctor. Decades later, through a strange series of events, he was recruited by the French Army as an emergency doctor liaison and deployed at the British Camp Bastion in Afghanistan, where he studied the British and American treatment for polytraumatized soldiers called Damage Control Resuscitation.

Back in France, Elie now works as an emergency doctor in the emergency services of Paris. He has a special interest in integrative medicine and works as an osteopath in private practice. He continues to work part-time in the UK National Health Service. He is also a composer of experimental music, and his triptych, *Antenatal, Coma,* and *DNA* will be released soon. *DNA* bears witness to his experience in Afghanistan. You can visit the author at www.eliepaulcohen.com

ABOUT THE TRANSLATOR

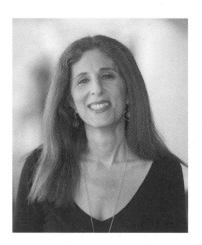

Jessica Levine is the author of *The Geometry of Love*, a Top 10 Women's Fiction Title in *Booklist* in 2015. She is also the author of *Nothing Forgotten: A Novel* and *Delicate Pursuit: Discretion in Henry James and Edith Wharton*. Her essays, short stories, and poetry have appeared in many publications including *The Southern Review* and *The Huffington Post*. She translates books from French and Italian into English.

Jessica holds a Ph.D. in English Literature from the University of California at Berkeley, where she was a Mellon Fellow. She was born in New York City and now lives in Northern California. You can find her at www.jessicalevine.com.

SELECTED TITLES FROM SPARKPRESS

SparkPress is an independent boutique publisher delivering high-quality, entertaining, and engaging content that enhances readers' lives. Visit us at www.gosparkpress.com

Engineering a Life, Krishan Bedi, $16.95, 9781943006434.
A memoir of Krishan Bedi's experiences as a young Indian man in the South in the 1960s, this is a story of one man's perseverance and determination to create the life he'd always dreamed for himself and his family, despite his options seeming anything but limitless.

The House that Made Me: Writers Reflect on the Places and People That Defined Them, edited by Grant Jarrett. $17, 978-1-940716-31-2.
In this candid, evocative collection of essays, a diverse group of acclaimed authors reflect on the diverse homes, neighborhoods, and experiences that helped shape them—using Google Earth software to revisit the location in the process.

A Story That Matters: A Gratifying Approach to Writing About Your Life, Gina Carroll, $16.95, 9-781-943006-12-0.
With each chapter focusing on stories from the seminal periods of a lifetime—motherhood, childhood, relationships, work, and spirit—*A Story That Matters* provides the tools and motivation to craft and complete the stories of your life.

Quiet the Rage: How Learning to Manage Conflict Will Change Your Life (and the World), Richard Burke, $22.95, 978-1-943006-41-0.
Where there are people, there is conflict—but conflict divides people. Here, expert Certified Professional Coach R.W. Burke helps readers understand how conflict works, how they themselves may actually be the source of the conflict they're experiencing in their lives, and, most important, how to stop being that source.

ABOUT SPARKPRESS

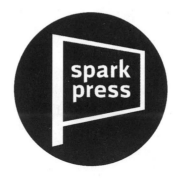

SparkPress is an independent, hybrid imprint focused on merging the best of the traditional publishing model with new and innovative strategies. We deliver high-quality, entertaining, and engaging content that enhances readers' lives. We are proud to bring to market a list of *New York Times* best-selling, award-winning, and debut authors who represent a wide array of genres, as well as our established, industry-wide reputation for creative, results-driven success in working with authors. SparkPress, a BookSparks imprint, is a division of SparkPoint Studio LLC.

Learn more at GoSparkPress.com